Eat for Life

99
HG/30/10

D0541256

About the Authors

Janette Marshall is editor of *BBC Good Health* magazine. She has been writing and broadcasting about food and health for more than ten years, and is well known as a contributor to national newspapers such as *The Independent* and *The Sunday Times*, and to leading magazines. As deputy editor of BBC Good Food she was responsible for several award-winning food and health features. She is also a committee member of the Guild of Food Writers.

Anne Heughan trained as a home economist and as a dietitian. Currently she is working for North East Thames Regional Health Authority as a regional co-ordinator for coronary heart disease. Previously she was assistant director of the Coronary Prevention Group, where she was responsible for campaigns on improving school meals and nutrition labelling. Anne has written many articles and books on food and health, and has also acted as a nutrition consultant for television and radio. She is a member of the British Dietetic Association, the Nutrition Society, the Royal Society of Medicine Forum on Food and Health, and the Faculty of Public Health Medicine Cardiovascular and Smoking Working Group.

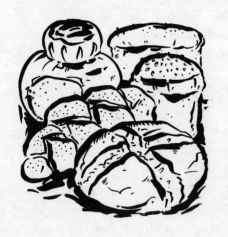

Eat for Life

The revolutionary

healthy eating plan

for all the family

**JANETTE MARSHALL
AND ANNE HEUGHAN**

ARROW

Published in 1992 by VERMILION
This revised edition published in 1993 by Vermilion Arrow
an imprint of Ebury Press
Random House UK Ltd
20 Vauxhall Bridge Road
London SW1V 2SA

A catalogue record for this book is available from the British Library.

ISBN 0 09 923001 1

EDITORS: Alison Wormleighton and Barbara Croxford
DESIGNER: Terry Jeavons
ILLUSTRATIONS: Ivan Hissey

Printed and bound in Great Britain
by Cox & Wyman Ltd, Reading, Berkshire.

WARNING
**If you have a medical condition, or are pregnant, the diet described
in this book should not be followed without first consulting your
doctor. All guidelines and warnings should be read carefully, and
the author and publisher cannot accept responsibility for injuries or
damage arising out of a failure to comply with the same.**

Contents

Foreword by
Professor Philip James

By changing what we eat, and taking regular exercise, we can substantially reduce our risk of heart disease and diet-related cancers. But for most people the most persuasive benefit of a change in diet and lifestyle is losing weight.

I spent five years as chairman of the World Health Organisation committee that published the report *Diet, nutrition and the prevention of chronic diseases*. During this time it became evident that there was a clear way to deal with weight control and the major, diet-related health problems of our times. The same diet that helps prevent heart disease can also be beneficial for avoiding coronary heart disease, diet-related cancers, dental decay, arthritis, osteoporosis – and weight control.

That world scientists have now arrived at this consensus is remarkable when considering that a body such as the WHO has to be conservative. It would be wrong to have ever-changing policies, but the evidence on diet was now not only strong but also longstanding, so a new policy on healthy eating was warranted. New evidence, however, is required to deal with the many unresolved issues.

We were able to recommend a set of nutritional goals which can encompass many different diets. Producing such a document is, however, of little relevance to improving Britain's poor record of diet-related disease and substantial increase in obesity, unless ordinary people are approached directly with the information, in an understandable form, needed to help them change their eating habits.

Motivating people to change is vital if we are going to improve our poor health record. It's estimated that one third of people in the UK are overweight. And if you consider that throughout your entire adult life you should not weigh more than your weight at the age of 25, then we have a real problem. As many as a quarter of us are already overweight by the age of 25, and thereafter most people gain more weight.

Overweight people are more likely to suffer coronary heart disease, high blood pressure, strokes, the commonest forms of diabetes, and diet-related cancers, such as breast cancer and cancer of the colon. Disability from hernia, arthritis and gallstones are also far commoner in the overweight. If we can help people to lose weight and preferably to prevent weight gain in adult life then we will go a long way to reducing the burden of ill health in Britain.

I welcome the publication of *Eat For Life*, which tackles the health problems head on. We need to prevent weight gain but also the many complications which arise from eating an inappropriate diet.

PHILIP JAMES, MA, DSC, FRCP, FRCP(E), FRSE
Director, Rowett Research Institute, Aberdeen,
October 1991.

Introduction to Eat for Life

Want to eat healthily? Need to lose weight? *Eat for Life* shows you how to do both – with just one way of eating.

Not since the *F-Plan Diet* has there been such a revolution. The world's leading scientists now agree that just a few simple changes to the way we eat will enable us to take the biggest step forward in healthy eating (and slimming) in the last twenty years.

So, if you have resisted making changes to the way you eat because you thought that experts could not agree, or that the advice they give is always changing: think again! No longer do you have to try to piece together the picture on healthy eating from a jigsaw of conflicting newspaper headlines. Scientists *do* now agree and *there is* a simple message about what makes a healthy diet. What's more, it doesn't cost the earth. Of course, there will still be silly, sensational headlines, and there will be new discoveries, but the information in *Eat for Life* is based on two scientific reports that incorporate all the studies of the last thirty years. So you can rely on it.

The message is simple. The healthiest people in the world follow three basic 'rules'. They eat:

1. About half their food as starchy food such as bread, pasta, rice or potatoes.
2. At least five portions of fruit and vegetables a day.

3. A minimum of saturated fat.

Eat for Life has incorporated this into:

- an Everyday 7-day 2,000 Calorie Eating Plan, for those who just want to follow a healthy diet
- a 28-day 1,200 Calorie Slimming Plan
- a 7-day 1,500 Calorie Slimming Plan
- an Easy Option Slimming Plan for busy people who want to slim.

All are suitable for men and women. There are no gimmicks – just good tasty food and menus that are low in fat, and as varied, or as predictable, as you want them to be.

Even if you don't follow the 28-day Slimming Plan you will soon discover that by following *Eat for Life* principles you will lose weight, if you need to. And you can stick with this way of eating, safely, for as long as you like.

Sounds too good to be true, but just one way of eating not only helps protect you and your family against heart disease, and diet-related cancers, but it can also help protect against other health problems such as:

- osteoporosis (thinning of the bones, leading to hip fractures and so on, later in life)
- high blood pressure
- gallstones
- some forms of diabetes
- tooth decay
- anaemia.

It also gives children the best start in life, helping to protect them against diseases which occur later in life, but which have their foundations laid by bad eating habits in childhood.

~ *Fit for Life* ~

From this it's obvious that eating well can certainly
do a lot to improve the quality of life, but diet alone
is not the answer. As coronary heart disease, for
example, has many causes, it is important to do
something about other risk factors, such as smoking,
raised blood pressure and lack of exercise.

Exercise is a necessary evil for some, fun for
others. Either way there is an impressive list of
benefits for regular aerobic exercise. In return for
three to five sessions a week you will:
- lose weight, if you need to
- improve your shape
- lower your risk of heart disease
- reduce stress
- feel less tired.

Whatever age you are, it's never too late to start.
Best of all, we should begin to exercise early in life
and continue through middle age and into old age, as
a part of weight control, and generally staying fit and
healthy. For an impressive list of the benefits of
exercise see the table in Appendix III, page 216.

Finally, adopting *Eat for Life*'s eating plans is not a
list of don'ts. It is one of the most positive things you
can do for yourself and your family.

PART ONE
The Healthiest Diet in the World

For most people, the main attraction of *Eat for Life* is that it shows you how to eat well. In addition, as we have seen in the introduction, it can also help protect you and your family against life-threatening diseases.

The basis of the healthiest diet in the world is:

1. Eat half your food as starchy foods such as bread, pasta, potatoes, cereals.
2. Eat at least 400 g/14 oz of fruit and vegetables a day, which adds up to five portions. And try to include 30 g/1 oz of pulses, nuts and seeds, especially if you are vegetarian.
3. Cut down on fat, particularly saturated fat.

Making these changes will revolutionise your meals and the way you shop. Instead of eating meat and two veg you will now be eating lots of potatoes, or pasta, or rice, plenty of vegetables and a minimum of lean meat or fish.

The way you shop will also change dramatically. Instead of first thinking which meat or fish to have for your main meal, your first thought is, 'Which starchy food will I build my meal around?' (For inspiration see the recipe section organised according to category of starchy foods.) You might choose bread or potatoes, rice, pasta or pulses. You could also serve bread with every meal like the French, Italians and other Mediterranean people. Incidentally, for everyday eating their bread is not spread with butter or margarine. Fruit, low-fat yogurt or a low-fat iced dessert, will replace the usual puddings. Adding more fruit and vegetables has never been easier because we now have such an array in our shops.

If you follow *Eat for Life* 'rules' you will be eating lots more fruit and vegetables and starchy fibre-rich foods. This will also help reduce the amount of fat in your diet – too much of which increases risk of heart disease and certain cancers. Cutting down on fat automatically helps you lose weight. This eating plan is also about eating less sugar, whether it is stirred into drinks, sprinkled on cereal or fruit, or hidden in cakes, sweets and other manufactured foods.

~ *What are starchy foods?* ~

Starchy foods are carbohydrate foods. There are two main types of carbohydrates:

Complex Carbohydrates (Starchy Foods)
Bread, pasta, potatoes, pulses, whole grains, other cereals, root vegetables such as sweet potatoes and cassava, and plantain. Dietary fibre has been isolated as a magic ingredient in previous diets, but we know that starchy foods, especially if they are wholemeal, are more valuable because they also contain more vitamins and minerals. All these nutrients work together to keep you healthy.

Free Sugars

This is the scientific name for what we usually call 'sugar'; refined from sugar cane or beet, bought by the packet, spooned from the sugar bowl, or eaten as a hidden ingredient in processed foods, cakes, biscuits and pastries. Free sugars also include glucose syrup, honey, concentrated fruit juices, and all the other names for sugar seen on food labels.

Scientists are now so confident about what makes up a healthy diet that they can tell us how much of each type of food we should eat. These amounts follow as *Eat for Life* Goals.

~ Eat for Life Goals ~
~ Starchy foods ~

Eat for Life Goal

For most people, reaching 50% means doubling the amount of bread, potatoes and cereals they eat. Fruit and vegetables are counted in this starchy food goal,

COMPLEX CARBOHYDRATES

UK TODAY   GOAL

27% calories from CC foods   **50**-70% calories from CC foods.

but because of their other valuable properties they also have a goal of their own (see page 15).

Contrary to popular belief, starchy foods like bread, potatoes and pasta are not fattening; it's the fat added during and after cooking that makes them 'fattening'. That's why chips are OK for treats, but not every day. As a rule we should eat boiled or steamed potatoes, rice, or other choices such as cous cous, bulghur wheat, buckwheat, pasta or noodles. Stir-frying, done quickly and with minimum oil, is fine occasionally.

Starchy foods are also more 'nutrient-dense' than free sugars. This means they contain more vitamins, minerals and trace elements per calorie (and per mouthful). In particular, they are rich in iron and B vitamins, and wholemeal versions are especially rich in essential fatty acids (EFAs), vitamin E and fibre.

Partly because of their fibre content, starchy foods are also filling. They are a much better choice for a snack than confectionery. So, instead of chocolate bars, let them eat cake (low-fat and fruit cakes without icing, wholemeal fruited buns and scones, teabreads and malt loaf), or sandwiches, toast, fancy breads.

~ Fibre ~

Eat for Life Goal
Around 27 g/1 oz is a realistic goal for most people, although you can go up to 40 g/$1^1/2$ oz. Fibre is found in food that comes from plants such as cereals, beans, peas, fruit, vegetables and pulses. Animal foods like meat, cheese, milk and eggs contain no fibre.

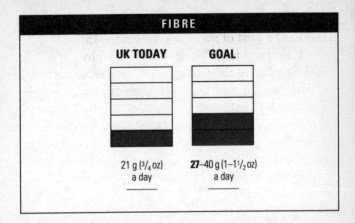

FIBRE

UK TODAY   GOAL

21 g (³/₄ oz)
a day

27–40 g (1–1¹/₂ oz)
a day

There is a recommended maximum because too much fibre in the form of raw bran can result in a loss of nutrients. Bran contains substances called phytates which reduce absorption of minerals like iron, zinc and calcium.

If you eat more fruit and vegetables and starchy foods, and take more exercise there should be no need to add bran to food. However, there's more to fibre than the constipation-conquering role of bran (found in wheat, maize and rice). The gummy type of fibre found in oats, beans, barley, rye, vegetables, and some fruit, called soluble fibre, also helps to lower blood cholesterol.

~ *Fruit and vegetables* ~

Eat for Life Goal
The 400 g (14 oz or nearly one pound) of fruit and vegetables a day excludes potatoes, which are counted as starchy foods. This adds up to about five

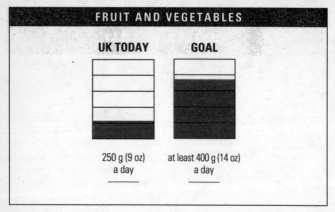

FRUIT AND VEGETABLES

UK TODAY   **GOAL**

250 g (9 oz)
a day

at least 400 g (14 oz)
a day

portions of fruit and vegetables a day. Don't panic, it isn't as odd as it sounds.

During a typical day you might have:

- a glass of fruit juice for breakfast – which equals one portion

- an apple or another piece of fruit as a snack during the day – each piece of fruit counts as one portion (see table, pages 17–18)

- at the main meal of the day two portions of vegetables (fresh, frozen or canned) excluding potatoes (see table on pages 18–20 for typical portion sizes)

- at one meal of the day you might have a fruit-based pudding, which counts as another portion.

In a normal day's healthy eating you will have met the target of five portions of fruit and vegetables. And if you can eat more, so much the better. If you don't eat meat or fish, try to include the 30 g (1 oz) a day of pulses, nuts and seeds.

PORTIONS OF FRUIT AND VEGETABLES – AIM FOR FIVE A DAY

FRUIT

Each of those listed equals 1 fruit portion, unless stated otherwise

Apple	
Avocado pear	$1/2$
Apricots, fresh or semi-dried	4
Banana	
Blackberries, raspberries, blackcurrants, cherries, gooseberries, stewed rhubarb and other cooked fruit	around 100 g ($3^1/2$ oz)
Clementine or other citrus such as mandarin, mineola, orange, satsuma, tangerine	
Damsons, greengages or other small plums	4
Dates, fresh or dried	4–6
Figs, fresh or dried	4
Grapefruit	$1/2$
Grapes	100 g ($3^1/2$ oz)
Kiwifruit	2
Mango	$1/2$
Melon	175 g (6 oz)
Nectarine	
Passion fruit	4–5

Pawpaw	1/2
Peach	
Pear	
Pineapple	75–100 g (3–3 1/2 oz)
Prunes	stewed: 6; semi-dried: 4
Sharon fruit	
Watermelon	200 g (7 oz)

FRUIT JUICE

1 citrus fruit squeezed	
200 ml (7 fl oz) glass fruit juice	
Individual carton fruit juice	

VEGETABLES

Portions are around 75–100 g (3–3 1/2 oz). Get to know how much this is in terms of 15ml tablespoonfuls. You can eat more, of course; the list is just a rough guide to give you an idea of the variety of vegetables available.

Artichoke, globe	
Asparagus spears	5
Baked beans	
Broad beans	30 ml (2 tbsp)
French and runner beans	
Beansprouts	120 ml (8 tbsp)

Broccoli and calabrese	2 medium–large spears
Brussels sprouts	9–10
Cabbage	
Carrots	30 ml (2 tbsp)
Cauliflower	8 florets
Celery	3 sticks
Chick peas	30–45 ml (2–3 tbsp)
Chinese leaf	2 large leaves
Coleslaw, low fat	30 ml (2 tbsp)
Corn on the cob	1 ear
Cucumber	5 cm (2 in) slice
Green banana	1/2
Leek	
Lentils	37–45 ml (2 1/2–3 tbsp)
Lettuce	16 leaves
Marrow	
Mushrooms, poached	10
Mustard and cress	1/2 punnet equals 1/4 portion
Okra	8 equal 1/4 portion
Onion	1 1/2–2
Parsnips	1 medium
Peas	45 ml (3 tbsp)
Pepper	
Plantain	1/3–1/2
Ratatouille	45 ml (3 tbsp)

Sauerkraut	45 ml (3 tbsp)
Spinach	
Swede	
Sweetcorn	
Tomatoes	1 large or 6 cherry
Turnip	
Watercress	1 bunch

~ Sugar ~

Eat for Life Goal
The aim is to at least halve your sugar consumption. The lower level of zero simply means that sugar is not needed in a healthy diet. When you eat starchy foods they are broken down to sugar (for energy), so you don't need to eat sugar itself, which contains no useful nutrients. Nevertheless, most people enjoy sweet things and don't want to give

SUGAR

UK TODAY   **GOAL**

15–20% calories
from sugar

No more than
10% calories
from sugar

HIDDEN SUGAR		
	Sugar	
	ml	tsp
Chocolate milk shake (1 glass)	55–100	11–20
Chocolate fudge cake (slice)	55	11
Cola (1 glass)	45	9
Mars-type bar	45	9
Chocolate digestive biscuit	10	2
Tomato soup (half a can)	5	1
Allbran cereal (1 bowl)	5	1
Coco Pops (1 bowl)	15	3
Plain ice cream (1 portion)	10	2
Fruit yogurt (one small carton)	15	3

them up entirely. If this is the case for you, one approach is to eat cakes and confectionery at weekends only, as a treat. Or, at least wean yourself off pudding with every meal, cookies with every coffee and Danishes with every drink. Cut down (with the aim of giving up) sugar in hot drinks; reduce the sugar content of your recipes; choose an alternative to sugar-coated breakfast cereals. And watch out for sugar in its other guises as sucrose, dextrose, glucose, fructose, maltose, honey, and so on.

~ *Fats* ~

In some countries people eat less than 30% of their calories as fat, but this amount would mean that the British diet would change drastically. While there's no harm in that, change takes time and a gradual process means you are more likely to stick to a lower-fat diet. Your tastes will also change, given time.

Cutting down on fat doesn't mean a fat-free diet. It's essential to eat some polyunsaturated fat, but too much fat, especially saturated fat, increases the risk of heart disease and heart attacks.

The reason for eating less fatty food, and more starchy food and more fruit and vegetables, is all to do with blood cholesterol. The higher the level of cholesterol in the blood the greater the risk of developing heart disease. High fat intake also increases the risk of some cancers.

Despite its bad reputation, cholesterol is essential for a healthy nervous system and for making hormones. The liver produces enough cholesterol for normal body functions, and it is carried in the bloodstream – hence the term blood cholesterol. Usually the body maintains its own balance, making more as it is needed and getting rid of excess, but sometimes the balance is upset.

If too many fatty foods are eaten, especially those containing saturated fats, there is a tendency for

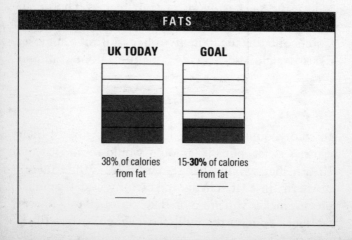

FATS

UK TODAY   **GOAL**

38% of calories   15-**30%** of calories
from fat   from fat

blood cholesterol to build up in the artery walls, making them narrower and slowing down the supply of blood to the heart, or even cutting it off completely, at which point a heart attack occurs.

Saturated Fats

Eat for Life Goal

Eating too much saturated fat can raise blood cholesterol levels and so increase the risk of heart disease. Saturated fats are found mainly in animal foods: fatty meat (such as belly pork, shoulder of lamb, mince, chops), suet, lard, dripping; and in dairy products such as full-fat (silver top) milk, butter, cream and high fat cheeses; in hard margarines and other cooking fats; in cakes, biscuits, pastry, puddings and chocolate.

SATURATED FATS

UK TODAY

GOAL

16% of calories from saturated fat

No more than 10% of calories from saturated fat

Polyunsaturated Fats

Eat for Life Goal

If the figures overleaf appear rather complicated, don't worry. They indicate that polyunsaturated fats help reduce blood cholesterol levels, but that you shouldn't eat lots of them on top of a diet already high in fat. The main thing is still to eat a low-fat diet, but make sure you eat some polyunsaturated fats (found in sunflower, corn, soya and other oils, fruits and vegetables), in place of saturated fats (see above) to ensure you receive enough essential fatty acids (EFAs), which the body cannot produce.

The oils in fish such as herring, mackerel and sardines contain a type of polyunsaturated fat that makes the blood less sticky, reducing the likelihood of heart attack and stroke. These oils are also vital for the development of the brain.

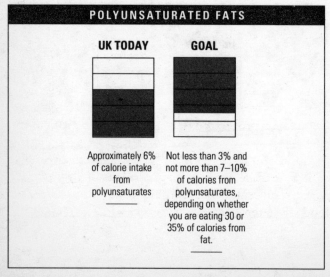

POLYUNSATURATED FATS

UK TODAY	GOAL
Approximately 6% of calorie intake from polyunsaturates	Not less than 3% and not more than 7–10% of calories from polyunsaturates, depending on whether you are eating 30 or 35% of calories from fat.

The upper limit was set because evidence suggests that eating too much polyunsaturated fat (at levels far higher than anything in a normal diet) might increase the risk of certain cancers. It's likely that if there are problems they are linked to existing disease and are not causing disease.

~ The Olive Oil Story ~

You may have heard that olive oil (rich in monounsaturates) is better for you than sunflower, soya and corn oils, which are rich in polyunsaturates. Like polyunsaturates, monounsaturates can help lower blood cholesterol levels, as part of a low saturated-fat diet.

So far it seems that in southern Italy and Greece, where a lot of olive oil is used, and little saturated fat is eaten, the rate of heart disease is very low, even though they eat as much fat as we do in Britain, where heart disease is rife.

However, the low rate of heart disease in the Mediterranean region could equally be due to low saturated fat intake, because less meat and almost no dairy produce is eaten. The Mediterranean diet is also rich in protective starchy foods and fruit and vegetables.

So, if you are thinking of switching to olive oil, use it to replace saturated fats. Priority is still to eat less fat, especially saturated fat, if we are to reduce blood cholesterol levels and the risk of heart disease.

~ *(M)eat to Live?* ~

You don't have to give up meat, and red meat, in particular, to have a healthy diet. Conversely, from the vegetarian perspective, you don't have to eat meat to be healthy.

For those who eat red meat, it is a good source of iron and zinc and contains a useful amount of B vitamins, especially vitamin B12, which is found almost exclusively in animal foods. For those who don't eat red meat, all these nutrients can be found elsewhere. However, iron and zinc are more efficiently used by the body in the form found in meat.

Zinc is found in wholemeal bread, pulses, eggs and nuts and iron in dark green vegetables, dried fruit, nuts, wholegrains and wholemeal bread. However, iron from these sources needs to be eaten with foods rich in vitamin C to make it usable by the body. This is not a problem, just something to be aware of if you don't eat meat, or if you are cutting down on it.

If you do like meat, eat meat, not fat. Pies, pâtés, sausages and some burgers are high in saturated fat. Better to eat meat less often and make sure it is lean than eat fatty meat (such as belly of pork, shoulder of lamb, mince, chops) every day. Better still, choose meat that has been produced organically and with proper consideration for animal welfare issues.

MEAT AND FISH

LOW-FAT meat and fish (in which 25% or less of the calories are from fat) MAY BE EATEN OFTEN

White fish, poached or steamed	Canned fish in brine
	Prawns
Roast chicken or turkey, without skin	Scallops
	Lean roast beef

MEDIUM-FAT meat and fish (in which 45% or less of the calories are from fat) MAY BE EATEN QUITE OFTEN

Grilled or steamed trout,	Stewed rabbit
Salmon	Lean roast leg of pork
Lean boiled ham	Lean roast venison
Lean roast duck, without skin	Stewed offal
Sardines and pilchards in tomato sauce	Lean grilled pork chop, without fat
	Stewed lean beef,

MEDIUM-HIGH FAT meat (in which around 60% of the calories are from fat) MAY BE EATEN RARELY AND IN SMALL QUANTITIES

Bacon	Salami
Mince	Luncheon meat
Chops	Pork pie and other meat pies
Gammon – meat and fat	Pâté
Liver sausage	Scotch eggs
Sausages	

Lean meat also includes game, which most people don't eat often. Like poultry it contains less fat then red meat. The fat is just under the skin so it can easily be cut away when preparing, or after cooking, before serving.

Eating fish twice a week instead of meat replaces saturated fats with unsaturated fats. White fish is low in fat and high in vitamins and minerals. Oily fish has the added advantage of being rich in essential fish oils, which make the blood less sticky and therefore less likely to clot and cause a heart attack. Obviously, to benefit, fish has to be a regular part of your diet.

Although shellfish are high in dietary cholesterol, the British seaside favourites, cockles and mussels, winkles and whelks, are low in fat – as are prawns, shrimps and crab – and are fine eaten regularly unless you have a high blood cholesterol.

CHOICE CHEESES

LOW-FAT cheese (in which 25% or less of the calories are from fat): fromage frais, quark and similar low-fat soft white cheeses

MEDIUM-FAT cheese (in which 45% or less of the calories are from fat): cottage cheese (35%)

HIGH-FAT cheese (in which 60% or more of the calories are from fat): Cheddar and other hard cheeses, blue cheeses, cream cheeses, Edam, Brie, Camembert, goat's cheese

Dairy products contribute calcium and protein – and a lot of fat. Choose low-fat versions of milk, cheese and yogurt, or, on special occasions, Greek yogurt instead of cream. And while eggs are nutritious and convenient, the general consensus is that four a week, including those in cooking, is enough. However, if you do not eat much saturated fat elsewhere in your diet, you might eat more.

~ Salt ~

Eat for Life Goal
The 12 g of salt that we eat each day is equivalent to $2^1/_2$ teaspoons. Only a fraction of the sodium (a component of salt) we eat is needed. Lowering sodium intake could reduce high blood pressure and heart disease, especially as there is a relationship between sodium intake and raised blood pressure as we increase in age.

SODIUM (SALT)	
UK TODAY	**GOAL**
12 g ('/₂ oz)/day sodium	Not more than 6 g ('/₄ oz)/day sodium

In fact, we could even halve the *Eat for Life* goal to 3 g a day (half a teaspoonful) without coming to any harm because all the salt you need (unless you are a lumberjack or working at the coalface, or in the desert) is in bread, cereals, fruit and vegetables. The reason most people get twice the amount they need is because they eat it unknowingly in processed foods and salty snacks.

~ *Protein* ~

There is no *Eat for Life* Goal for protein because, generally speaking, as long as enough calories are eaten, enough protein is obtained. Even in countries where cereals and pulses are the main foods eaten (which they are by the majority of the world's population) those who have enough to eat have enough protein. We often forget that even vegetables provide protein because we usually think of it in terms of meat, fish, cheese and eggs.

Vegetarian protein
It used to be thought that vegetarians had to combine at the same meal foods from two or three of the four basic groups of vegetarian protein foods.
The vegetarian groups of protein are:
- beans and pulses
- nuts and seeds
- cereals and grains
- milk, cheese and yogurt.

Now we know this is unnecessary. However, it is a good idea for vegetarians (and meat-eaters, alike) to eat different sources of protein — it is unwise to be over-reliant on any one food. For example, vegetarians can easily eat too much saturated fat if they rely heavily on cheese and eggs for protein

~ Alcohol ~

Eat for Life Goal

There's no 'need' to drink any alcohol! If you don't drink, you can eat more without putting on weight. Some studies have suggested that drinking could be good for you at low levels of around 10–20 g of alcohol a day, which is about 1–1$\frac{1}{2}$ units of alcohol (a couple of glasses of wine or just under one pint of beer). People who drink that much may have a reduced risk of heart disease and cholesterol gallstone formation. On the other hand, there are a lot more studies that point out the health risks associated with drinking.

Because most adults do drink, 'safe' levels have been set. They are lower for women because alcohol

---

ALCOHOL

UK TODAY

GOAL

8% of calories from alcohol

No more than 4% of calories from alcohol

stays longer in women's bodies and is more concentrated. Women become drunk faster than men drinking the same amount of alcohol and they feel the effects for longer.

Even if you don't drink much, the advice is: *Don't drink it all at once.* Spread out drinks so that you have one or two alcohol-free days each week. Also, spread out the drinks during a session, interspersing them with non-alcoholic drinks.

Although the body detoxifies alcohol (which is, in fact, a toxin or poison) drinking can leave you short of B vitamins, vitamin C and minerals. Unfortunately, alcohol does not come complete with the vitamins and minerals needed. And, because it is a diuretic (stimulates urination), it causes further losses of vitamins. Like sugar, the only thing alcohol offers as food is calories. So not only will it go to your head, but also to your waistline.

'Safe' levels are:

- not more than 21 units of alcohol a week for men
- not more than 14 units of alcohol a week for women.

As a general rule, one unit of alcohol equals the following:

- 1 single pub measure ($1/6$ th gill/25 ml) of spirits, or 25 ml (1 fl oz)
- 1 small (79 ml/$2^3/4$ fl oz) glass of sherry or other fortified wine
- 1 small (125 ml/4 fl oz) glass of wine
- $1/2$ pint (300ml/10 fl oz) ordinary beer, lager or cider

- $1/4$ pint (125 ml/4 fl oz) strong beer, lager or cider
- 2 small (125 ml/4 fl oz) glasses of low alcohol wine
- $1^1/2$ pints (900 ml/30 fl oz) low alcohol beer, lager or cider
- Scottish pub spirit measures are 1.2 units

This is useful as a general guide, but it can be misleading because some wines, beers and spirits are stronger than others.

Pregnancy

During pregnancy (and before conception), it is best to avoid alcohol as it can be passed from the mother's bloodstream to the baby through the placenta and so put an unborn child at risk. And even moderate amounts can affect conception. One study shows that as little as two pints of beer a day reduces sperm formation.

The greatest risk to babies is during the early weeks of pregnancy when the baby's brain is developing.

In America, there are government warnings (similar to those on cigarette packs in Britain) on alcoholic drinks. The government warns: (1) According to the Surgeon General women should not drink alcoholic beverages during pregnancy because of the risk of birth defects; (2) Consumption of alcoholic beverages impairs your ability to drive a car or operate machinery, and may cause health problems.

~ *Eating Enough Vitamins and Minerals* ~

Everyone needs vitamins and minerals on a daily basis. Some need more than others. And the $64,000 question for most people is: How much of each vitamin or mineral do I need? Individual prescriptions can only be worked out after many scientific tests; and, for most people, this is not necessary. Just as vitamin pills are not necessary. With a few exceptions, such as a woman's folic acid and iron needs in pregnancy, vitamins and minerals should be obtained from food and not from pills.

One reason for caution about vitamin and mineral pills is that vitamins probably act together with other substances in food, such as fibre, minerals and possibly as-yet-unknown substances. These additional ingredients are unlikely to be in vitamin pills. Taking vitamin pills can also upset the natural balance. For example, in food the B vitamins are invariably found in clusters, so taking B vitamins individually as vitamin supplements may upset some body processes, or create extra requirements. This might be as harmful as not eating enough vitamins. All the more reason to eat well.

Although each vitamin and mineral is important, there is a lot of scientific interest in three vitamins in particular: beta-carotene (which the body turns into vitamin A), and vitamins C and E. These often occur in clusters in fruit and vegetables, and beta-carotene is the pigment that gives green, yellow and orange fruits their colour. All three are have protective antioxidant powers.

The importance of antioxidants is their ability to

neutralise 'free radicals', which are highly active and damaging. Free radicals may start off some cancers and heart disease. They are produced through natural body processes, but they can also be created by pollutants, such as chemicals, cigarette smoke and radiation (i.e., X-rays).

Although free radicals exist only momentarily, they need to be dealt with because inside cells they are capable of damaging DNA, the genetic material in cells, which can produce potentially carcinogenic (cancer-causing) cells. And they may set up chain reactions in the arteries that increase the risk of heart attack.

Antioxidant vitamins such as vitamin A, in the form of beta-carotene, vitamin C and vitamin E inactivate free radicals and so prevent their destructive effects.

Although there are government figures on how much of each vitamin and mineral the average person probably needs, it is enough to be aware of the different vitamins and minerals, the foods in which they are rich, and to eat them regularly. Such foods are listed below.

ACE Nutrients

Vitamin C is widely available in fruit and vegetables, and should be eaten daily. **Good sources** include: blackcurrants, guava, dark green vegetables, lemons, oranges and orange juice, other citrus fruit, strawberries, grapefruit and grapefruit juice, mango, spinach, melon, paw paw (papaya), and other fruit and vegetables.

Vitamin E. The amount you need depends on how much polyunsaturated fat you eat; vitamin E is needed to help your body use polyunsaturates (it actually prevents them from being oxidised and forming harmful free radicals). **Good sources** include: vegetable oils (sunflower, soya, corn, peanut, olive), blackberries, nuts, eggs, asparagus, tuna in oil, avocado, muesli, wholemeal bread, brown rice, salmon and some margarines.

Beta-carotene. Widely available in fruit and vegetables, there is some evidence that beta-carotene is protective against cancer through its antioxidant powers. **Good sources** are: carrots, spinach, sweet potatoes, spring greens, watercress, broccoli, canteloupe melon, liver, pumpkin, apricots, tomatoes, peaches and mango.

Vitamin A. This vitamin is needed for maintenance of a healthy skin and surface tissues. Eating too much vitamin A over a period of time may be dangerous as it can lead to liver and bone damage, especially in children and pregnant women. Taken in high doses preconceptually or by women who are pregnant, vitamin A can also cause birth defects in unborn babies (see page 38). **Good sources** are: Liver, butter and margarine, cheese, eggs, carrots, spinach, sweet potatoes, spring greens and oily fish.

The B Group

The B vitamins found in starchy foods, whole grains, meat and milk, are also vital for health – in particular, the maintenance of the nervous system, and the release of energy from food during digestion.

Vitamin B1 (Thiamin) is needed to turn food into energy. The amount required depends on the amount of food eaten. **Good sources** are: yeast extract, brown rice, nuts, pork, cod's roe, bulghur wheat, peas, lentils, wholemeal pasta and bread, and fortified breakfast cereals.

Vitamin B2 (Riboflavin). Like thiamin, riboflavin is needed for energy release. For sedentary people, the recommended amount depends on the number of calories eaten; active people need more. **Good sources** are: yeast extract, liver, ox heart, eggs, fish roe, fortified breakfast cereals, green leafy vegetables, pulses, lentils and lean meat.

Vitamin B3 (Niacin) is also involved in the release of energy, with the amount needed depending on the calories eaten. The body can also produce its own niacin from some protein foods. **Good sources** include: yeast extract, nuts, liver, oily fish, bacon, chicken, turkey, sardines (canned in oil), fortified breakfast cereals, wholemeal bread and brown rice.

Vitamin B6. The amount of vitamin B6 needed is related to protein intake. Despite popular belief, oral contraceptives do not increase the need for B6, nor does pregnancy or breastfeeding. **Good sources** are: yeast extract, oats, plantain, fish, liver, bacon, brown rice, bananas, green leafy vegetables, fortified breakfast cereals and wholemeal bread.

Vitamin B12 is needed to help protect the nerves and to prevent anaemia. In particular, B12 works with folic acid. High intakes of this vitamin are not dangerous. Vegetarians and vegans need to pay attention to intake, as B12 is found in animal produce. **Good sources** are: liver, kidney, sardines (canned in oil), mackerel and other oily fish, cod's roe, red meat, white fish, chicken, eggs, cheese, yogurt, milk, oysters and rabbit.

Folates is the name given to a group of substances made from folic acid. Pregnant women need extra folates. New evidence shows that folic acid supplements taken before and during the first three months of pregnancy can prevent spina bifida in babies among women who have already had a pregnancy affected by neural tube defects. All women who are likely to become pregnant would benefit from eating more foods rich in folic acid.

Although liver is a rich source of folic acid, the Department of Health has advised women who may become pregnant not to eat it, because it might contain too much vitamin A, which can cause deformities in unborn babies (see page 36). Animal feed supplemented with too much vitamin A caused the problem; as this fat soluble vitamin is stored in the liver, it can build up to toxic levels. However, once the feed problem is resolved this will no longer be a problem. **Good sources** are: liver, green leafy vegetables such as spinach, spring greens, Brussels sprouts, pulses, lentils, nuts, kidney, wholemeal bread, citrus fruit, eggs, brown rice, fruit (fresh and dried) and fortified breakfast cereals.

Vitamin D. Although we talk about 'vitamin D', it is in fact a hormone that is needed for the absorption of calcium, which is in turn essential for bones and teeth. It is also called the 'sunshine vitamin' because most vitamin D is made in our skin by the action of the sun – not sunbathing, just natural daylight. Vitamin D is found in only a few foods, yet it is vital for the development of strong teeth and bones because it is needed for calcium and phosphorus absorption. Toddlers and children who don't eat enough may develop rickets. Those mainly at risk are members of the Asian community, whose traditional diet is low in calcium and who have limited exposure to daylight. Deficiency can also lead to osteomalacia (softening of the bones from lack of vitamin D in adults, similar to rickets). **Good sources** are: mackerel, herring, kipper, salmon (canned), sardines (canned), pilchards (canned), tuna (canned in oil), brown rice, eggs, milk, butter and margarine (all types are fortified by law).

Minerals

Calcium. More than 90% of bone is laid down during growth and most of the calcium in the body is found in bones and teeth. Bone mass peaks between the ages of thirty and forty and then begins to decline. In women, this process accelerates at the menopause, with the risk of osteoporosis, in which the bones become so fragile that half of all women suffer a hip fracture by the time they are seventy. However, high doses of calcium, especially around the menopause, are not recommended. There could be some evidence that eating calcium-rich foods or taking low doses of calcium supplements may reduce bone loss. Scientists are still gathering that evidence. Eating well throughout life and taking enough exercise, and not smoking, are the best protection against calcium-deficiency related diseases. **Good sources** include: sprats, canned fish, spinach, cheese, such as Cheddar and Edam, low-fat milk, yogurt, eggs and custard.

Iron is essential for red blood cells and most is recycled by the body, although some is lost by bleeding. Anaemia (shortage of haemoglobin, the oxygen-carrying pigment of the red blood cells) is caused by an iron deficiency, and most at risk are adolescents and menstruating women. Tannin in tea can also inhibit the absorption of iron. It's estimated that about 10% of women may need supplementary iron tablets. Pregnant women with low iron stores may need tablets, too, but most healthy mothers do not need extra as menstrual loss will not be adding to needs. **Good sources** are: liver (see page 38), other offal, sprats, cockles (boiled), winkles and other shellfish, dried fruit such as apricots, peaches and prunes, bulghur wheat, sardines (and other oily canned fish), fortified breakfast cereals, wholemeal bread, pulses and lean meat.

Zinc is vital for several body systems and for building cells. The body is quite good at conserving zinc. Absorption increases in pregnancy so there should be no extra requirements. **Good sources** are: liver, lamb, rump steak (and other types of beef), bacon, oysters, lean pork, shrimps (boiled), turkey (roast, dark meat), ox heart (stewed), sardines (canned), breakfast cereals, cheese, wholemeal bread, rye bread, fish and pulses.

Potassium. Adequate intake of potassium helps to prevent high blood pressure, as well as enabling nerves and muscles to function. **Good sources** are: all fruit and vegetables, nuts, breakfast cereals, herring and other types of oily fish.

Selenium is an enzyme which helps prevent cell damage that might initiate cancer or heart disease. Too much selenium can be harmful, so stick to the dosages suggested on dietary supplements. Levels in wheat, grain and therefore bread, and also dairy produce, depend on levels in the soil and vary regionally. **Good sources** include: liver and other organ meats, white fish and shellfish, red meat, brown rice, prawns, muesli, wholegrain cereals, milk, eggs and wholemeal bread.

~ *The* Eat for Life *Shopping Basket* ~

It's a popular view that no single food is either healthy or unhealthy. It's the sum total of the *diet* that is either healthy or unhealthy. However, some foods contribute more to healthy living and eating than others, and should feature more often in the *Eat for Life* shopping basket. No matter how super a food, no one food contains all nutrients. That's why it's important to eat plenty of different foods.

That said, many fruits, vegetables, and starchy foods contain special combinations or clusters of vitamins and minerals that are associated with a lower risk of heart disease and some diet–related cancers.

What we eat now	What we should eat
Bread, cereal, pasta, potatoes	**more, switch** to mostly wholemeal
Cakes, biscuits	**less, switch** to mostly wholemeal
Meat, fresh	**less, switch** to lean only
Meat products: sausages, pies, pâtés, pasties	**occasionally**, stick to low-fat versions
Fish, white and oily	**more**, of both types
Fruit and vegetables	**more**
Pulses	**more**
Milk	**switch** to skimmed or semi-skimmed
Cheese, mainly hard	**switch** to mainly low-fat
Butter	**less**
Margarine	**less, switch** to those high in polyunsaturates or low-fat spreads
Oils	**less, switch** to those high in either polyunsaturates or monounsaturates
Eggs	**stay same**, present level is four a week
Sugar and confectionery	**less**, or cut out
Alcohol	**stick to safe levels**

~ The Healthy Eating Pyramid ~

The pyramid shows that the foundation of a healthy diet is starchy food and fruit and vegetables. On top of this, in smaller amounts, are low-fat dairy produce, lean meat, fish, nuts and eggs. And on the very top, in the smallest amounts, are sugar, butter, margarine and fatty foods.

Drinks aren't shown, but thirst is best quenched with water. Fruit juices and skimmed milk are a good choice, if you like milk as a drink. Go easy on caffeine-containing coffee, tea and colas – find some herb or fruit tea alternatives for some drinks during the day (check with your doctor if you are pregnant). And, watch the amount of alcohol you drink.

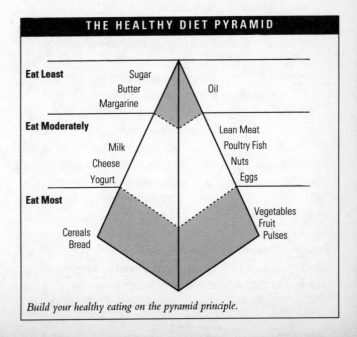

THE HEALTHY DIET PYRAMID

Eat Least Sugar / Butter / Margarine Oil

Eat Moderately Milk / Cheese / Yogurt Lean Meat / Poultry Fish / Nuts / Eggs

Eat Most Cereals / Bread Vegetables / Fruit / Pulses

Build your healthy eating on the pyramid principle.

PART TWO
Lose weight Once and for All

~ The Perfect Slimming Diet ~

Unlike low-calorie and crash diets, *Eat for Life*'s 28-day Slimming Plan is based on a realistic 1,200 calories a day. In addition there is a 1,500 Calorie Plan for those who still want to lose weight but at a slower rate. This in itself is a revolution, reflecting the latest thinking on dieting that shows:

- You are more likely to stick to a plan with 1,200 or 1,500 calories, therefore you are more likely to succeed
- You will find it more filling, satisfying and pleasant to follow
- While your weight loss will be marginally slower, it will be more permanent.

Twelve hundred or 1,500 calories a day might sound a lot, if you are used to crash diets of 600, 800 or even the usual 1,000 calories a day. While slimming on crash diets might make you lose weight quickly, you put it all back on again after the diet. The only way to stay the right weight *permanently* is to *Eat for Life*.

Here's an example of the weight loss you might expect. If you ate 2,000 calories a day before the 28-day Slimming Plan, after a week you will have lost 5,600 calories, the equivalent of $1^1/2$ lb or 0.7 kg of fat. With water loss during the first week, that could amount to as much as a 6^1/$_2$ lb or 2.9 kg of weight loss.

After that you can expect to lose a further 1^1/$_2$ lb or 0.7 kg of fat a week – and more if you exercise regularly. In 28 days you could lose about a stone. This is not crash dieting. Weight loss at such a moderate speed is permanent, provided you continue to follow *Eat for Life*'s basic 'rules' and eat half your calories as starchy food, plus five portions of fruit and vegetables a day, with a minimum of fat, especially saturated fat.

Adopting these rules will lead to a gradual weight loss for those who have pounds to shed. But, if you want to do it slightly more quickly – or you simply like to have the menus and recipes worked out for you – then in this section of *Eat for Life* you will find the slimming plan to suit you.

Eat for Life positively encourages you to eat because it is now understood that on a diet rich in starchy foods, like bread and pasta, and fruit and vegetables, you don't have to go hungry or suffer food cravings. To be slim you have to change permanently the way you eat. So there is absolutely no point going on a crash diet or a slimming diet that you can't live with. Instead, *Eat for Life* shows you how to eat to be slim for life.

Eat for Life: **An Executive Summary**

Briefly, your diet should be comprised of the following four components:
- Half the diet should be starchy foods like cereals, breads, potatoes, rice and other grains

- You should eat at least five portions (14 oz/ 400 g) of fruit and vegetables a day, especially green and yellow fruit and vegetables, and citrus fruit
- The rest of your diet includes small amounts of lean meat or low-fat dairy produce. Make a meal of fish twice a week, instead of meat (animal food is, however, optional and a matter of personal choice)
- Go easy on the alcohol, salt and sugar.

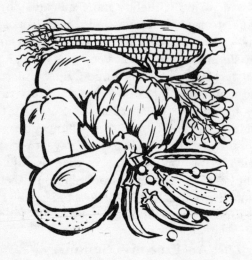

~ The 28-day Slimming Plan ~

1,200 calories per day

The *Eat for Life* slimming plans fulfil the goals of 50% calories from starchy foods; not more than 30% calories from fat. And they're low in saturated fat, sugar and salt.

Daily allowance

300 ml (1/2 pint) skimmed milk for tea and coffee
    or 150 ml (1/4 pint) skimmed milk and 150 ml
    (5 fl oz) low-fat natural yogurt
    or 200 ml (7 fl oz) soya milk
15 g (1/2 oz) low-fat spread
    or 7 g (1/4 oz) polyunsaturated margarine
    or 10 ml (2 tsp) French dressing (see page 205)
    or 5 ml (1 tsp) unsaturated oil
A portion of fresh fruit.

Bread, Rice and Pasta

Where these items are specified in the lunch or dinner menus, use the following guidelines for portion sizes.
Bread Instead of 2 large thick slices of wholemeal bread 100 g (31/2 oz), you can use 2 large thick slices of brown, Granary or white bread or 1 large pitta bread or 75 g Ciabatta or 1 large bap.
Rice 50 g (2 oz) uncooked rice = 100 g (31/2 oz) cooked rice
Pasta 50 g (2 oz) uncooked pasta = 100 g (31/2 oz) cooked pasta

Dieting tips

- Vegetables should not be tossed in butter, margarine or low-fat spread before serving.
- Keep the use of oil or fat in cooking to a minimum, especially for stir-fried vegetables or browning of meat.
- All spices must be fried before adding any liquid to help develop their flavour, with the exception of those used in marinades.
- Eat larger portions of vegetables if you are hungry.

Note: If you find dieting difficult because you need to snack throughout the day, it is better to eat some fresh fruit or salad as a snack, and then eat the potato, rice, remaining salad and protein part of the meal at the proper time.

PORTIONS OF FRUIT	
1 apple	3 apricots
1 small banana	large slice melon
1 orange	125 g (4 oz) raspberries
1 pear	3 plums
10 strawberries	10 grapes
1 peach	

BREAKFASTS

WEEK 1

Monday

1 glass fresh orange juice
1 large, thick slice wholemeal toast
scraping of low-fat spread
10 ml (2 tsp) marmalade or jam or
lemon curd

Tuesday

1/2 grapefruit
45 ml (3 tbsp) bran flakes and milk
from allowance

Wednesday

Apple sliced and mixed with
45 ml (3 tbsp) unsweetened muesli
milk from allowance

Thursday

1 glass fresh orange juice
1 wholemeal muffin
scraping of low-fat spread
yeast extract

Friday

Banana, sliced and mixed with
45 ml (3 tbsp) bran flakes
milk from allowance

—————————— *Saturday* ——————————

1 glass fresh orange juice
1 large, thick slice Granary bread
1 small slice lean ham
or 1 small cheese triangle

—————————— *Sunday* ——————————

$^1/2$ grapefruit
1 large, thick slice wholemeal toast
mushrooms cooked 10 g ($^1/3$ oz) low-fat spread in
non-stick pan.

WEEK 2

—————————— *Monday* ——————————

2 wholewheat biscuits with 15 ml (1 tbsp) raisins
milk from allowance

—————————— *Tuesday* ——————————

1 glass fresh orange juice
1 large, thick slice wholemeal toast
1 triangle cheese spread

——————————*Wednesday*——————————

$^1/2$ grapefruit
40 g ($1^1/2$ oz) porridge oats made with water
milk from allowance
10 ml (2 tsp) brown sugar or honey

----------------------------- *Thursday* -----------------------------

1 glass fresh orange juice
1 wholemeal hot-cross bun – warmed in the
microwave or toasted
scraping of low-fat spread

----------------------------- *Friday* -----------------------------

1 banana
1 large thick slice wholemeal toast
10 ml (2 tsp) Citrus Spread (p. 20)

----------------------------- *Saturday* -----------------------------

1 glass fresh orange juice
45 ml (3 tbsp) muesli mixed with
a chopped apple
milk from allowance

----------------------------- *Sunday* -----------------------------

$1/2$ grapefruit
1 large, thick slice wholemeal toast
1 poached or boiled egg
scraping of low-fat spread

WEEK 3

----------------------------- *Monday* -----------------------------

1 glass fresh orange juice
45 ml (3 tbsp) unsweetened muesli
milk from allowance

Tuesday

$1/2$ grapefruit
1 large, thick slice wholemeal toast
scraping of low-fat spread
yeast extract

Wednesday

45 ml (3 tbsp) bran flakes
1 banana, sliced
milk from allowance

Thursday

1 glass fresh orange juice
1 wholemeal hot-cross bun
scraping of low-fat spread

Friday

1 apple
1 wholemeal muffin
scraping of low-fat spread
10 ml (2 tsp) marmalade or jam
or lemon curd

Saturday

1 glass orange juice
1 slice wholemeal toast
2 halves grilled tomatoes
50 g (2 oz) mushrooms cooked in a
scraping of low-fat spread

Sunday

$^1/_2$ grapefruit
1 slice wholemeal toast
1 rasher grilled back bacon
Vegetarian option: 1 poached egg

WEEK 4

Monday

1 glass fresh orange juice
40 g ($1^1/_2$ oz) porridge oats made with water
milk from allowance
10 ml (2 tsp) brown sugar or honey

Tuesday

1 banana
1 large, thick slice wholemeal toast
scraping of low-fat spread
10 ml (2 tsp) marmalade or jam
or lemon curd

Wednesday

45 ml (3 tbsp) muesli mixed with
1 chopped apple
milk from allowance

Thursday

1 glass fresh orange juice
1 wholemeal muffin
scraping of low-fat spread
10 ml (2 tsp) marmalade or jam
or lemon curd

--------------------------- *Friday* ---------------------------

1 apple
2 wholewheat biscuits
milk from allowance

--------------------------- *Saturday* ---------------------------

1 glass fresh orange juice
1 poached egg on one large slice wholemeal toast
scraping of low-fat spread

--------------------------- *Sunday* ---------------------------

1 glass fresh orange juice
sliced tomato and cheese on toast

LUNCHES

*Page numbers following a dish indicate the page on which
the recipe appears.*

WEEK 1

--------------------------- *Monday* ---------------------------

50 g (2 oz) lean roast chicken meat and Italian Salad
(p.173) sandwich made with 2 large, thick slices
wholemeal bread
1 apple
Vegetarian option: 1 hard-boiled egg, sliced,
and Italian Salad (p.173) sandwich made with 2 large,
thick slices wholemeal bread
1 apple

—————————————— *Tuesday* ——————————————

175 g (6 oz) jacket potato filled with 150 g (5 oz)
baked beans and 25 g (1 oz) lean ham and
chopped tomato salad
1 banana
Vegetarian option: 175 g (6 oz) jacket
potato filled with 150 g (5 oz) baked beans and 15 g
(^{1}/2 oz) Parmesan cheese and chopped tomato salad
1 banana

—————————————*Wednesday*—————————————

Mexican Tuna (p.122) salad sandwich made with 2
large, thick slices Granary bread and
an extra tomato
1 orange
Vegetarian option: 50 g (2 oz) Hummus (p.153)
salad sandwich made with 2 large, thick slices of
Granary bread
1 orange

—————————————— *Thursday* ——————————————

50 g (2 oz) reduced–fat hard cheese and salad
sandwich made with a large brown bap
1 pear

—————————————— *Friday* ——————————————

175 g (6 oz) jacket potato with 75 g (3 oz) cottage
cheese, grated carrots and 15 g (^{1}/2 oz) nuts
1 portion fresh fruit salad

─────────────── *Saturday* ───────────────

Black Bean Soup (p.153)
1 wholemeal roll
1 apple

─────────────── *Sunday* ───────────────

100 g (3^1/2 oz) lean roast leg of lamb
Ratatouille (p.130), peas
100 g (3^1/2 oz) cooked basmati rice
Fruit Kebabs (p.193)
Vegetarian option: 50 g (2 oz) reduced-fat hard
cheese with 100 g (3^1/2 oz) cooked basmati rice,
Ratatouille (p.130), peas
Fruit Kebabs (p.193)

WEEK 2

─────────────── *Monday* ───────────────

150 g (5 oz) vegetarian pizza
tomato and pepper salad
1 pear

─────────────── *Tuesday* ───────────────

50 g (2 oz) lean ham, and Winter Salad (p.175)
sandwich made with 2 large, thick slices
wholemeal bread
1 apple
Vegetarian option: 50 g (2 oz) Hummus (p.153)
and Winter Salad (p.175) sandwich made with
2 large, thick slices wholemeal bread
1 apple

—————————— *Wednesday* ——————————

50 g (2 oz) sardine and tomato sandwich made with
2 large, thick slices wholemeal bread
1 orange
Vegetarian option: cucumber Raita (p.201) and
Bean Salad (p.158) and pitta bread
1 orange

—————————— *Thursday* ——————————

175 g (6 oz) jacket potato filled with 50 g (2 oz)
reduced-fat hard cheese and grated carrot
1 apple

—————————— *Friday* ——————————

Pan Bagnet: Niçoise (p.123)
sandwich made with a large piece
of French bread
1 banana
Vegetarian option: Niçoise (p.123)
sandwich made with a large piece
of French bread
1 banana

—————————— *Saturday* ——————————

Avocado, Prawn and Celery Salad (p.182)
1 wholemeal roll
cherries
Vegetarian option: Avocado, Walnut
and Celery Salad (p.182)
1 wholemeal roll
cherries

Sunday

---

75 g (3 oz) roast chicken, no skin
175 g (6 oz) boiled potato
broccoli
carrots
Fresh Fruit (p.186) Platter with Mango Sauce (p.195)
Vegetarian option: 1 portion Lazy Lentils (p.152)
150 g (5 oz) boiled potatoes
broccoli
carrots
Fresh Fruit Platter (p.186) with Mango Sauce (p.195)

WEEK 3

Monday

Toasted sandwich made with 50 g (2 oz) reduced-fat
grated cheese and 2 large, thick slices wholemeal
bread and salad
1 banana

Tuesday

---

3 oz (75 g) chicken and Turkish Salad (p.174)
sandwich, made with 2 large, thick slices
of Granary bread
1 pear
Vegetarian option: peanut butter and
Turkish Salad (p.174) sandwich made with 2 large,
thick slices of Granary bread
1 pear

Wednesday

50 g (2 oz) Aubergine Pâté (p.169)
with wholemeal pitta bread
tomato and cucumber salad
1 apple

Thursday

Egg and Watercress salad (p.123)
sandwich made with 2 large, thick
slices wholemeal bread
1 peach

Friday

50 g (2 oz) Smoked Mackerel Pâté (p.122)
with 2 large, thick slices wholemeal toast
Fennel, Apricot and Walnut Salad (p.173)
1 apple
Vegetarian option: 50 g (2 oz) Bean Pâté (p.156)
with 2 large, thick slices wholemeal toast
Fennel, Apricot and Walnut Salad (p.173)
1 apple

Saturday

Chicken and Blue Cheese Toasted
Sandwich.(p.124) and salad
grapes
Vegetarian option: Toasted Sandwich (p.124)
made with 40 g (1 1/2 oz) blue cheese instead
of chicken
grapes

Sunday

75 g (3 oz) lean roast pork
red cabbage
175 g (6 oz) boiled new potatoes
green beans
small portion Cheesecake (p.194)
with Rhubarb Sauce (p.196)
Vegetarian option: Leek Risotto (p.135)
green beans
small portion Cheesecake (p.194)
and Rhubarb Sauce (p.196)

WEEK 4

Monday

Crab and Lemon Coleslaw (p.177) sandwich made
with 2 large, thick slices wholemeal bread
1 apple
Vegetarian option: 50 g (2 oz) Hummus (p.153)
with Lemon Coleslaw (p.177) sandwich made with
2 large, thick slices wholemeal bread
1 apple

Tuesday

50 g (2 oz) lean roast beef with Italian Salad (p.173)
and 5 ml (1 tsp) horseradish sandwich made with
2 large, thick slices wholemeal bread
1 nectarine
Vegetarian option: Black Bean Soup (p.153) with
2 large thick slices wholemeal toast and
Italian Salad (p.173)
1 nectarine

———————— *Wednesday* ————————

50 g (2 oz) prawns with Winter Salad (p.175)
in 1 wholemeal pitta bread
1 orange
Vegetarian option: 150 g (5 oz) vegetarian
wholemeal pizza and Winter Salad (p.175)
1 orange

———————— *Thursday* ————————

Chicken and Tabbouleh Sandwich (p.125) made
with 2 large, thick slices wholemeal bread
1 banana
Vegetarian option: Tabbouleh (p.125) sandwich
made with 25 g (1 oz) chopped nuts instead
of chicken, and 2 large, thick slices wholemeal bread
1 banana

———————— *Friday* ————————

Wholemeal Pasta Salad (p.139) with green salad
3 plums
Vegetarian option: Wholemeal Pasta Salad (p.139)
made with 50 g (2 oz) reduced-fat cheese per person
instead of crab, with green salad
3 plums

———————— *Saturday* ————————

Pasta, Bean and Vegetable Soup (p.140) and
a wholemeal roll, served with
15 g ($^1/_2$ oz) Parmesan cheese
$^1/_2$ sliced orange and $^1/_2$ sliced banana

———————— *Sunday* ————————

100 g (3^1/2 oz) roast beef
175 g (6 oz) boiled potatoes
cabbage
carrots
Walnut Stuffed Pears (p.192) with
15 ml (1 tbsp) Greek yogurt
Vegetarian option: Chick Pea Hot Pot (p.130)
175 g (6 oz) boiled potatoes
cabbage
carrots
Walnut Stuffed Pears (p.192) with
15 ml (1 tbsp) Greek yogurt

EVENING MEALS

WEEK 1

———————— *Monday* ————————

Butterbean and Mushroom Bake (p.151)
175 g (6 oz) jacket potato
grated carrot salad
tomato salad
1 glass fresh orange juice

———————— *Tuesday* ————————

Chicken with Watercress Sauce (p.172)
100 g (3^1/2 oz) cooked pasta
broccoli
carrots
Pears with Fresh Ginger (p.189)

Vegetarian option: 1 Stuffed Pepper (p.162)
broccoli
carrots
a bread roll
Pears with Fresh Ginger (p.189)

Wednesday

100 g (3¹/₂ oz) cooked Spicy Rice (p.131)
100 g (3¹/₂ oz) fish or chicken tikka kebab made
with 100 g (3¹/₂ oz)
Yogurt Tandoori Marinade (p.196)
Turkish Salad (p.174)
lettuce
1 fresh mango
Vegetarian option: 225 g (8 oz) Vegetable
Chilli (p.155)
100 g (3¹/₂ oz) cooked Spicy Rice (p.131)
Turkish Salad (p.174)
lettuce
1 fresh mango

Thursday

Pasta with Tomato and Aubergine Sauce (p.144)
mixed salad
1 scoop Lemon Sorbet (p.183)

Friday

100 g (3¹/₂ oz) boiled rice
Stir-fry Vegetables (p.160) made with
75 g (3 oz) pork
baked apple with raisins and
low-fat yogurt from allowance

Vegetarian option: Stir-fry Vegetables (p.160) with
25 g (1 oz) flaked toasted almonds
100 g (3^1/2 oz) boiled rice
baked apple and raisins and
low-fat yogurt from allowance

———————— *Saturday* ————————

175 g (6 oz) boiled new potatoes
Green Beans in Tomato Sauce (p.168)
100 g (3^1/2 oz) baked salmon
Peach Brûlée (p.188)
Vegetarian option: Spinach and Cheese
Squares (p.165)
175 g (6 oz) boiled new potatoes
Green Beans in Tomato Sauce (p.168)
Peach Brûlée (p.188)

———————— *Sunday* ————————

50 g (2 oz) Bean Pâté (p.156) and pitta bread
with green salad
grapes

WEEK 2

———————— *Monday* ————————

Vegetable and Fish Kebab (p.166)
175 g (6 oz) boiled potatoes
broccoli
raspberries and ^{1}/2 banana
Vegetarian option: Pepper and Potato (p.167)
75 g (3 oz) boiled potatoes

broccoli
carrots
raspberries and $^1/_2$ banana

--------------------- *Tuesday* ---------------------

Keema (p.150)
100 g ($3^1/_2$ oz) cooked boiled rice
carrot salad
tomato salad
1 apple
Vegetarian option: Spinach and
Lentil Dhansak (p.170)
100 g ($3^1/_2$ oz) cooked boiled rice
carrot salad
tomato salad
1 apple

--------------------- *Wednesday* ---------------------

Pasta with Liver (p.146)
fennel and tomato salad
1 slice fresh pineapple
Vegetarian option: 100 g ($3^1/_2$ oz) cooked
pasta with spicy tomato sauce
(Tomato sauce (p.200) heated with 1 dried chilli)
fennel and tomato salad
1 slice fresh pineapple

--------------------- *Thursday* ---------------------

75 g (3 oz) lean roast chicken
Indian Potatoes (p.128)
carrots

peas
Fresh Fruit Platter (p.186)
Vegetarian option: Chick Pea Hot Pot (p.130)
Indian Potatoes (p.128)
carrots
peas
Fresh Fruit Platter (p.186)

Friday

grilled 175 g (6 oz) trout
175 g (6 oz) boiled potatoes
peas
baked tomatoes with herbs
Fruit Parcels (p.187)
Vegetarian option: Courgette and
Bean Goulash (p.154)
175 g (6 oz) boiled potatoes
peas, tomatoes
Fruit Parcels (p.187)

Saturday

grilled 100 g ($3^1/2$ oz) pork chop, trimmed of fat,
with Red Pepper Sauce (p.202)
175 g (6 oz) boiled potatoes
Poppy Seed Leeks (p.168)
carrots
1 scoop Strawberry Yogurt Ice Cream (p.185)
Vegetarian option: Pasta with
Green Beans and Mushrooms (p.143)
Poppyseed Leeks (p.168)
carrots
1 scoop Strawberry Yogurt Ice Cream (p.185)

Sunday

Pasta al Funghi (p.142)
green salad
Dried Fruit Salad (p.189)

WEEK 3

Monday

Nasi Goreng (p.132)
tomato and cucumber salad
sprouted lentil salad or green salad
3 plums
Vegetarian option: Nasi Goreng (p.132)
without the meat but served with an omelette
(using 1 egg per person)
tomato and cucumber salad
sprouted lentil salad
3 plums

Tuesday

grilled tuna steak
Tomato Salsa (p.202)
carrot salad
1/4 of a large baguette
Fruit Kebabs (p.193)
Vegetarian option: Hungarian Potatoes (p.130)
carrot salad
1/4 of a large baguette
Fruit Kebabs (p.193)

Wednesday

grilled chicken
(marinaded in Soy Sauce Marinade (p.198) if desired)
100 g (3¹/₂ oz) Lemon Rice (p.136)
Green Beans in Tomato Sauce (p.168)
sweetcorn
blackberries and apple

Vegetarian option: Green Beans in
Tomato Sauce (p.168)
100 g (3¹/₂ oz) Lemon Rice (p.136) with
25 g (1 oz) chopped cashews
sweetcorn
Raita (p.201)
blackberries and apple

Thursday

Kedgeree (p.137)
tomato salad
Bean Salad (p.158)
kiwi fruit
Vegetarian option: Leek Risotto (p.135)
Bean Salad (p.158)
tomato salad
kiwi fruit

Friday

Pork and Bean Goulash (p.154)
175 g (6 oz) jacket potato
green beans
1 scoop Rhubarb Sorbet (p.183)

Vegetarian option: Courgette and
Bean Goulash (p.154)
175 g (6 oz) jacket potato
green beans
1 scoop Rhubarb Sorbet (p.183)

--- *Saturday* ---

Spicy Lamb with Chick Peas and Apricots (p.149)
(replace chicken with lamb in chick pea,
chicken and apricot dish)
100 g (3^1/2 oz) Persian Rice (p.137)
Turkish Salad (p.174)
green salad
Pears with Fresh Ginger (p.189)
Vegetarian option: Spicy Chick Peas
and Apricots (p.149)
100 g (3^1/2 oz) Persian Rice (p.137)
Turkish Salad (p.174)
green salad
Pears with Fresh Ginger (p.189)

--- *Sunday* ---

Salad Niçoise (p.181)
Granary bread
1 apple
Vegetarian option: Vegetarian Salad Niçoise
(p.181) (made without the tuna)
Granary bread
1 apple

WEEK 4

--------------------------- *Monday* ---------------------------

Fish Stew (p.207)
1 bread roll
mixed salad
1 slice fresh pineapple
Vegetarian option: Lentil and
Spinach Soup (p.157)
1 bread roll
mixed salad
1 slice fresh pineapple

--------------------------- *Tuesday* ---------------------------

grilled home-made hamburger,
with Tomato Sauce (p.200) (optional)
100 g (3^1/2 oz) Spicy Rice (p.131)
green salad
carrot salad
baked banana with yogurt from allowance
Vegetarian option: Mange Tout and Carrots
with Soy Sauce (p.161)
100 g (3^1/2 oz) Spicy Rice (p.131)
green salad
carrot salad
baked banana with yogurt from allowance

--------------------------- *Wednesday* ---------------------------

Seafood Salad (p.178)
bread roll
cucumber salad
tomato salad

melon and strawberries
Vegetarian option: Spinach and
Cheese Squares (p.165)
1 bread roll
cucumber salad
tomato salad
melon and strawberries

--- *Thursday* ---

100 g (3^1/2 oz) roast pork
175 g (6 oz) boiled potatoes
Italian Cabbage (p.167)
peas
peaches and raspberries
Vegetarian option: Butterbean and
Mushroom Bake (p.151)
175 g (6 oz) boiled potatoes
Italian Cabbage (p.167)
peas
peaches and raspberries

--- *Friday* ---

Spicy Chicken Noodles (p.147)
Garden Salad (p.176)
Mango and Tomato Salsa (p.203)
fresh fruit salad
Vegetarian option: Spicy Noodles (p.147)
made with 25 g (1 oz) chopped peanuts
instead of the chicken
Garden Salad (p.176)
Mango and Tomato Salsa (p.203)
fresh fruit salad

Saturday

Seafood Risotto (p.133)
Watercress and Orange Salad (p.175)
Mushroom Salad (p.174)
Peaches Stuffed with Almonds (p.190)
Vegetarian option: Courgette Risotto (p.135)
Watercress and Orange Salad (p.175)
Mushroom Salad (p.174)
Peaches Stuffed with Almonds (p.190)

Sunday
---

150 g (5 oz) vegetarian pizza
Carrot and Nut Salad (p.176)
tomato salad
1 slice of pineapple

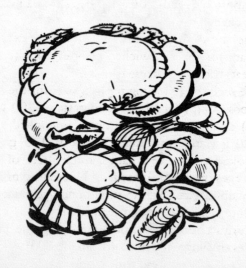

~ Easy Option Slimming Plan ~

If there never seems to be enough time in the day to do everything that needs to be done – let alone think about losing weight – then the Easy Option Plan is designed with you in mind. All you need to do is choose one of the breakfasts, one of the lunches and an evening meal. If you prefer to eat breakfast mid-morning instead of first thing, that is entirely up to you. Although you could eat pasta and tomato sauce every night, we wouldn't recommend it! Any diet is much healthier and more nutritious if you vary it as much as possible.

Although we haven't stated portion sizes we would suggest the following:

1. Use large thick slices of bread for sandwiches and breakfast.
2. Choose reduced-fat hard cheeses instead of high-fat cheeses
3. Use the minimum amount of filling, except for salad, for the sandwiches – about 50 g (2 oz) of meat, fish pâté, cheese or egg.
4. We used the following portion sizes for the starchy foods: 50 g (2 oz) uncooked pasta or 100 g (3 1/2 oz) cooked pasta; 50 g (2 oz) uncooked rice or 100 g (3 1/2 oz) cooked rice or 175 g (6 oz) cooked potato or 2 large, thick slices of bread. Try to use wholemeal varieties as much as possible, but that doesn't mean you can't use white rice, pasta or bread.
5. Always choose lean meat and keep the portion sizes small.

Daily allowance

300 ml ($^1/_2$ pint) skimmed milk
  or 150 ml (5 fl oz) skimmed milk and 150 ml
  (5 fl oz) low-fat yogurt.
  or 200 ml (7 fl oz) soya milk
15 g ($^1/_2$ oz) low-fat spread
  or 5 ml (1 tsp) oil
  or 7.5 ml ($^1/_2$ tbsp) French dressing (see
  page 205)
  or 7 g ($^1/_4$ oz) polyunsaturated margarine
A portion of fresh fruit.

BREAKFAST

1 slice wholemeal toast and scraping low-fat spread
from allowance and 1 small slice lean ham and
1 portion fruit

1 slice granary toast and 1 triangle cheese spread and
1 portion fruit

45 ml (3 tbsp) bran flakes and milk from allowance
and 1 portion fruit

2 Weetabix and milk from allowance and
1 portion fruit

2 Shredded Wheat and milk from allowance and
1 portion of fruit

1 slice wholemeal toast and 10 ml (2 tsp) peanut
butter and 1 portion fruit

45 ml (3 tbsp) muesli and milk from allowance and
1 portion fruit

1 wholemeal hot-cross bun and scraping low-fat
spread from allowance and
1 portion fruit

1 slice brown bread and scraping low-fat spread from
allowance and 1 portion fruit

1 slice wholemeal bread and scraping low-fat spread
from allowance and 10 ml (2 tsp) jam or marmalade
or lemon curd and
1 portion of fruit

1 slice rye bread and 2 halves grilled tomato and
50 g (2 oz) mushrooms cooked in
2.5 ml ($^1/2$ tsp) low-fat spread from allowance and
1 portion fruit

40 g (1$^1/2$ oz) porridge oats made with water,
10 ml (2 tsp) brown sugar, milk from allowance and
1 portion fruit

1 slice wholemeal bread, scraping low-fat spread from
allowance and 1 poached egg and 1 portion fruit

1 wholemeal muffin and scraping low-fat spread from
allowance and 10 ml (2 tsp) jam or marmalade or
lemon curd and
1 portion fruit

LUNCH

Small slice vegetarian pizza and
1 portion fruit

Cheese and salad sandwich and
1 portion fruit

Roast beef and horseradish and salad sandwich and 1
portion of fruit

Roast chicken and Italian Salad (p.173) sandwich
and 1 portion of fruit

Hummus (p.153) and salad and pitta bread
and 1 portion fruit

Egg and Watercress Sandwich (p.123)
and 1 portion fruit

Pasta, Bean and Vegetable Soup (p.140) and
1 wholemeal roll and 1 portion fruit

Tomato and Courgette Soup (p.171) and 1 bread roll
and reduced-fat cheese and
1 portion fruit

Ham and salad sandwich and 1 portion fruit

Sardine, tomato and lettuce sandwich
and 1 portion fruit

Niçoise salad (p.123) sandwich
and 1 portion fruit

Peanut butter and salad sandwich and
1 portion fruit

Smoked Mackerel Pâté (p.122) and salad and
pitta bread and 1 portion fruit

Aubergine Pâté (p.169) and pitta bread, salad
and 1 portion fruit

40 g ($1^{1}/2$ oz) blue cheese and tomato toasted
sandwich, salad and 1 portion fruit

Curried chicken toasted sandwich, made with
50 g (2 oz) lean roast chicken,
10 g ($1/3$ oz) reduced-fat mayonnaise, 10 g ($1/3$ oz)
low-fat yogurt, 2.5 ml ($1/2$ tsp) jam and
a pinch of curry powder; salad and
1 portion fruit

Prawns and Winter Salad (p.175) and
75 g (3 oz) Ciabatta and
1 portion fruit

Pork and Cabbage salad (p.124) sandwich
and 1 portion fruit

Mexican Tuna (p.122) and salad sandwich
and 1 portion fruit

Summer Soup (p.127) and 1 bread roll,
cheese salad and 1 portion fruit

Jacket potato with cottage cheese and grated carrots
and 25 g (1 oz) nuts and
1 portion fruit

Jacket potato with baked beans and salad
and 1 portion fruit

Jacket potato with small portion chilli con carne and
salad and 1 portion fruit

Jacket potato with cheese and salad
and 1 portion fruit

Jacket potato with Provençale Sauce (Tomato Sauce
(p.200) and 50 g (2 oz) prawns cooked together) and
salad and
1 portion fruit

Jacket potato with Ratatouille (p.130)
and 1 portion fruit

Cheese and Turkish Salad (p.174) sandwich
and 1 portion fruit

Chicken and Tabbouleh (p.125) sandwich
and 1 portion fruit

Salad Niçoise (p.181) and 1 bread roll
and 1 portion fruit

Thai Chicken (p.180) Salad and 1 bread roll
and 1 portion fruit

Broad bean, cheese, pepper and lettuce salad
and 1 bread roll and 1 portion fruit

Spinach and Ham Salad (p.179) and 1 granary roll
and 1 portion fruit

Brown Rice Salad (p.134) and 1 portion fruit

Bean Salad with Tuna (p.158) and 1 bread roll
and 1 portion fruit

Sardines on toast (2 large slices) and salad
and 1 portion of fruit

Tuna mixed with sweetcorn and chopped celery
on toast (2 large slices) and
1 portion of fruit

Jacket potato with ham mixed with sweetcorn,
fennel, red pepper and
10 ml (2 tsp) French Dressing (p.205)
and 1 portion of fruit

40 g (1$^{1}/_{2}$ oz) blue cheese, chopped apple,
celery and lettuce sandwich and
1 portion of fruit

Grated cheese and grated carrot sandwich and
1 portion of fruit

Salmon and yogurt mixed with chopped mint
and salad sandwich and
1 portion of fruit

Beef and grated beetroot and apple sandwich and
1 portion of fruit

25 g (1 oz) cottage cheese and 25 g (1 oz) blue
cheese mixed together and salad sandwich and
1 portion of fruit

150 g (5 oz) baked beans on toast (2 large slices)
and salad and 1 portion of fruit

Quarter of small avocado, mashed and salad sandwich
and 1 portion of fruit

Egg and salad roll and 1 portion of fruit

Marinated herring and beetroot and apple salad with
1 roll and 1 portion of fruit

EVENING

Rice with Keema (p.150) and 2 salads
and 1 portion fruit

Pasta with Bolognaise sauce and 2 salads
and 1 portion fruit

Rice and stir-fried liver and 2 vegetables
and 1 portion fruit

Rice with chicken tikka and 2 salads
and 1 portion fruit

Pasta with Tomato and Aubergine Sauce (p.144) and
mozzarella cheese and 1 salad and 1 portion fruit

Boiled potatoes and 100 g ($3^1/2$ oz) grilled pork
chop with the fat removed and
2 vegetables and 1 portion fruit

Jacket potato and chicken with large portion
Stir-fry Vegetables (p.160) and
1 portion fruit

Rice with beef and Stir-fry Vegetables (p.160) and
1 salad and 1 portion fruit

Pasta with Provençale sauce (Tomato Sauce (p.200)
and prawns and cod) and 1 salad
and 1 portion fruit

Rice with Ratatouille (p.130) and cheese and
1 salad and 1 portion fruit

Pasta with small portion Tomato Sauce (p.200)
cooked with mushrooms and pork chop and
1 salad and 1 portion fruit

Boiled potatoes with lemon chicken (small breast of
chicken cooked in Lemon Marinade (p.196))
and 2 vegetables
and 1 portion fruit

Pasta with Red Pepper Sauce (p.202) and
15 g (^{1}/2 oz) Parmesan cheese and salad
and 1 portion fruit

Spicy Rice (p.131) with 75 g (3 oz) lean leg of lamb
and vegetable kebab and 1 vegetable
and 1 portion fruit

Boiled potatoes with grilled trout and 2 vegetables
and 1 portion fruit

Pasta with Kidney Beans and Bacon (p.141)
and 2 salads and 1 portion fruit

Boiled potatoes with 3 grilled fish fingers and
2 vegetables and
1 portion of fruit

Boiled potatoes with grilled fish cakes (2) and
2 vegetables and
1 portion of fruit

Tuna and Potato Bake (p.129) and 2 vegetables
and 1 portion fruit

Boiled potatoes, 100 g (3^1/2 oz) grilled rump steak
and 2 salads and 1 portion fruit

Rice with Stir-fry Vegetables (p.160) and
15 g (^{1}/2 oz) flaked almonds and
25 g (1 oz) reduced-fat hard cheese, grated,
and 1 portion fruit

Pasta with Courgette and
Bean Goulash (p.154) and 1 salad
and 1 portion fruit

Boiled potatoes, 125 g (4 oz) baked salmon
and 2 vegetables and 1 portion fruit

Rice with Ratatouille (p.130), 75 g (3 oz) lean
roast leg lamb and 1 vegetable
and 1 portion fruit

Chick Pea Hot Pot (p.130) and rice and 2 salads
and 1 portion fruit

Rice, 125 g (4 oz) grilled hamburger and
2 salads and 1 portion fruit

Jacket potato, Lazy Lentils (p.152) and 2 salads
and 1 portion fruit

Hungarian Potatoes (p.130), 100 g (3^1/2 oz) grilled
pork chop with the fat removed and 2 vegetables and
1 portion fruit

Pasta with Green Beans and Prawns (p.143)
and 1 salad
and 1 portion fruit

Leek Risotto (p.135) and 2 salads
and 1 portion fruit

Pasta al Funghi (p.142) and 2 salads
and 1 portion fruit

Rice with small chicken breast cooked in
Red Pepper Sauce (p.202) and 1 salad
and 1 portion fruit

Boiled potatoes, Spicy Fish Tikka and 2 salads
and 1 portion fruit

Jacket potato, 100 g (3^1/$_2$ oz) grilled leg of lamb with
the fat removed and 2 vegetables and
1 portion of fruit

Boiled potatoes, 75 g (3 oz) roast chicken, no skin,
and 2 vegetables and 1 portion fruit

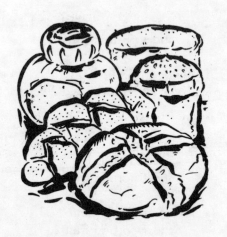

USING MANUFACTURED FOODS

Sometimes, preparing food can seem like too much effort, particularly when you are trying to diet. To help you diet the Easy Option Plan allows you to choose an occasional ready-made meal as an alternative to cooking. However, some of these dishes are higher in fat and more expensive than food prepared at home, so we certainly don't suggest that you use them all the time.

LUNCH

Try to choose a sandwich made from thick-cut bread and filled with plenty of salad; always have a piece of fruit. Here are a selection of sandwiches made by various manufacturers that contain approximately 300 calories or less.

Boots Shapers:
Smoked ham, soft cheese and pineapple with lettuce – 212 Calories
Turkey and Chinese leaf with sage and onion mayonnaise – 242 Calories
Cheese and celery with mayonnaise – 265 Calories
Chicken and Chinese leaf and lemon mayonnaise – 242 Calories
Tuna, mayonnaise and cucumber – 202 Calories
Prawn, apple and celery with mayonnaise – 270 Calories
Soft cheese, celery, sweetcorn and red peppers – 227 Calories

Poached Scotch salmon and Chinese leaf with mayonnaise – 260 Calories
Barbecue chicken with smoky barbecue mayonnaise and lettuce – 265 Calories
Chicken Korma, apricot, almonds and Chinese leaf – 281 Calories

Sainsbury's:
Red salmon and cucumber – 281 Calories
Chicken salad – 271 Calories
Ham and tomato – 281 Calories
Mixed summer salad with fromage frais and chives – 214 Calories
Cottage cheese and Florida salad – 275 Calories

Tesco:
Healthy Eating ham salad – 242 Calories
Healthy Eating chicken and Chinese leaf – 253 Calories
Healthy Eating prawn cocktail – 245 Calories
Healthy Eating chicken Waldorf – 295 Calories
Healthy Eating tuna and cucumber – 270 Calories
Oak-smoked ham with salad – 283 Calories

Marks and Spencer:
Prawn and cocktail sauce – 242 Calories
Danish ham and salad – 240 Calories
Tandoori chicken – 268 Calories
Fresh chicken with lemon mayonnaise – 234 Calories

Safeway:
Salmon and cucumber – 310 Calories
Country salad – 305 Calories

Honey roast ham salad – 215 Calories
Smoked ham, soft cheese and pineapple – 240 Calories
Tandoori pitta – 300 Calories

Asda:
Roast chicken and salad – under 300 Calories
Tuna – under 300 Calories
Bacon, tomato and lettuce – under 300 Calories
Roast ham and turkey – under 300 Calories
Roast chicken – under 300 Calories

Waitrose:
Salmon and cucumber sandwich – 275 Calories
Club sandwich – 301 Calories
Prawn cocktail sandwich – 282 Calories

EVENING

Ready-made meals have revolutionised many of our lives. No longer is the sole choice between cooking foods at home or eating out. We can now eat ready-made meals that require minimal preparation. However, research has shown that if we eat these dishes we may not eat vegetables with them. In line with the *Eat for Life* principles, you should try to have at least two vegetables or salads with your main meal and a piece of fruit to meet the daily target. So choose a ready-made meal with no more than 450 Calories – including rice, pasta or potato. If the ready-made meal doesn't include rice, pasta or potato, and is under 300 Calories per serving, you can add your own.

All Calories are per serving of the ready-made meal.

Asda:
Frozen meals
Chicken and ham lasagne – under 300 Calories
Plaice Mexicana – under 300 Calories
(Add 175g (6oz) boiled potatoes)
Chicken Mandarin – under 300 Calories
(Add 100g (3¹/₂oz) boiled rice)

Chilled
Chicken biryani – under 450 Calories
Pasta and tuna bake – under 450 Calories
Vegetable cannelloni – under 450 Calories
Chicken korma and rice – under 450 Calories
Beef stew and dumplings – under 450 Calories
Chicken supreme with rice – under 450 Calories
Chicken chow mein – under 450 Calories

Sainsbury's:
Frozen meals
Healthy Cuisine lean beef lasagne – 375 Calories
Healthy Cuisine spinach and ricotta cannelloni –
363 Calories
Healthy Cuisine chicken Madras with turmeric
rice –358 Calories
Healthy Cuisine glazed chicken with rice –
328 Calories
Spaghetti Bolognaise – 415 Calories
Cappelletti Milanese – 430 Calories
Prawn curry and rice – 367 Calories

Chilled meals
Mushroom and ricotta cheese cannelloni –
410 Calories
Chicken korma with turmeric rice – 270 Calories
Spicy chicken fajitas – 357 Calories
Tagliatelle vegetali – 300 Calories
Fisherman's pie – 253 Calories
Cottage pie – 296 Calories
Chilli beef enchiladas – 345 Calories
Vegetable lasagne – 241 Calories
Bangers and mash – 325 Calories
Jacket potato with chicken and broccoli –
307 Calories

Tesco:
Frozen
Healthy Eating plaice with wine, mushroom and
 prawn sauce – 279 Calories
(Add 175 g (6 oz) boiled potatoes)
Healthy Eating chicken tikka masala with rice –
367 Calories
Healthy Eating sweet and sour chicken and rice –
316 Calories
Healthy Eating Kasmiri korma with rice –
319 Calories
Healthy Eating ocean pie – 269 Calories
Healthy Eating cod mornay with vegetables –
258 Calories (Add 175 g (6 oz) boiled potatoes)
Healthy Eating vegetable chilli with rice –
272 Calories

Chilled meals
Vegetable casserole with dumplings – 241 Calories
Healthy Eating chicken casserole with dumplings –
284 Calories
Healthy Eating lasagne – 339 Calories
Chicken korma with rice snack pot – 292 Calories

Microwave meals
Tuna lasagne – 384 Calories
Lancashire hot pot – 282 Calories
Beef stew with dumplings – 306 Calories

Birds Eye:
Healthy Options honey-glazed chicken with white
and wild rice – 420 Calories
Healthy Options Kashmiri beef curry with basmati
rice – 410 Calories
Healthy Options chicken in red wine with vegetable
rice – 320 Calories
Healthy Options beef Cantonese with noodles –
240 Calories
Healthy Options vegetable lasagne al forno –
300 Calories
Healthy Options spaghetti Bolognaise – 420 Calories
Healthy Options chicken chasseur with rice –
440 Calories
Gino Ginelli pizza quattro with ham, mushrooms and
sweetcorn – 315 Calories
Birds Eye seafood and chicken paella – 335 Calories
Birds Eye prawn curry with rice – 370 Calories
Birds Eye beef stew and dumplings – 350 Calories

Findus:
Lean Cuisine glazed chicken with rice – 272 Calories
Lean Cuisine chicken and prawn Cantonese with rice – 272 Calories
Lean Cuisine lamb tikka masala with rice – 256 Calories
Lean Cuisine vegetable risotto – 300 Calories
Lean Cuisine spicy chicken creole with rice – 286 Calories
Lean Cuisine zucchini lasagne – 315 Calories
Lean Cuisine chilli con carne with rice – 420 Calories
Lean Cuisine fisherman's pie – 320 Calories

Heinz:
Weight Watchers pasta shells with vegetables and prawns – 225 Calories
Weight Watchers vegetable curry and rice – 286 Calories
Weight Watchers chicken Marengo and rice – 272 Calories
Weight Watchers Quorn chow mein – 202 Calories
Weight Watchers vegetable cannelloni – 212 Calories
Weight Watchers mushroom pasta bake – 285 Calories
Weight Watchers beef Oriental with special egg rice – 281 Calories
Weight Watchers cauliflower cheese with potato – 258 Calories
Weight Watchers seafood lasagne – 231 Calories
Weight Watchers French bread pepperoni pizza – 243 Calories

Boots:

Microwave meals

Shepherd's pie – 250 Calories

Shapers ham and mushroom lasagne – 282 Calories

Shapers tuna and pasta bake – 246 Calories

Shapers chicken supreme – 255 Calories

Shapers chicken curry and rice – 263 Calories

Frozen

Shapers beef lasagne – 299 Calories

Salmon mornay – 299 Calories (Add about 175 g
(6 oz) boiled potatoes)

Chicken and asparagus bake – 294 Calories
(Add potatoes, as above)

Cod and prawn bake – 275 Calories
(Add potatoes, as above)

Vegetable gratin – 290 Calories
(Add potatoes, as above)

Marks and Spencer:

Layered vegetable loaf – under 300 Calories
(Add 175 g (6 oz) boiled potatoes)

Chicken Jalfrezi – 253 Calories
(Add 100 g (3^1/2 oz) boiled rice)

Vegetable pasta bake – 294 Calories

Prawns with spring onion and ginger – 138 Calories
(Add 100 g (3^1/2 oz) boiled rice)

Filled plaice mornay – 194 Calories (Add 6 oz
(175 g) boiled potatoes)

Cod Florentine – under 300 Calories (Add 175 g
(6 oz) boiled potatoes)

Chicken with cashew nuts – 127 Calories (Add 100 g
(3^1/2 oz) boiled noodles)

Chicken tarragon – 253 Calories (Add 175 g (6 oz) boiled potatoes)
Chilli con carne – 273 Calories (Add 100 g (3^1/$_2$ oz) boiled rice)
Chicken and prawn creole – under 300 Calories (Add 100 g (3^1/$_2$ oz) boiled rice)
Ham tagliatelle snack – under 300 Calories
Vegetable chilli – under 300 Calories (Add 100 g (3^1/$_2$ oz) boiled rice)
Bacon and mushroom snack jacket – under 300 Calories

Safeway:
Frozen
Hot pot – 320 Calories
Lamb and apple bake – 420 Calories
Chinese style stir-fry – 240 Calories (Add 100 g (4 oz) boiled rice)
Vegetable Dhansak with pilau rice – 450 Calories
Prawn Gobi masala with spiced basmati rice – 405 Calories
Roast beef platter – 385 Calories
Cauliflower cheese – 380 Calories

Chilled
American-style jambalaya – 355 Calories
Vegetable stir-fry with beef – 225 Calories (Add 100 g (4 oz) boiled rice)
Vegetable chilli – 180 Calories (Add 100 g (4 oz) boiled rice)
Ratatouille – 190 Calories (Add 100 g (4 oz) boiled rice)
Moussaka – 355 Calories

Tagliatelle with tuna and sweetcorn – 385 Calories
Beef enchiladas – 385 Calories
Creole gumbo pot – 220 Calories (Add 100 g (4 oz)
boiled rice)

Microwave meals
Pasta Bolognaise – 273 Calories
Beef stew with dumplings – 303 Calories

Co-op:
Microwave meals
Vegetable lasagne – 225 Calories
Tagliatelle carbonara – 366 Calories
Beef stew and dumplings with scalloped potatoes –
431 Calories
Beef lasagne – 375 Calories
Vegetable curry – 225 Calories (Add 100 g (3^1/2 oz)
boiled rice)

Frozen
Beef curry with rice – 449 Calories
Chilli con carne and rice – 357 Calories
Spaghetti Bolognaise – 364 Calories
Chicken curry with rice – 398 Calories
Vegetable curry and rice – 252 Calories
Cauliflower cheese – 174 Calories (Add 175 g (6 oz)
boiled potatoes)

Waitrose:
Chilled
Penne Arabiata – 302 Calories
Chicken tikka noddles – 311 Calories
Shepherd's pie – 331 Calories

Lamb Dhansak – 290 Calories (Add 100 g (3^1/2 oz) boiled rice)
Cannelloni di carne – 432 Calories
Vegetarian Shepherd's pie – 279 Calories

Frozen
Sweet and sour chicken with egg-fried rice – 406 Calories
Chilli prawns with rice – 283 Calories
Chicken chow mein – 322 Calories
Vegetable lasagne – 334 Calories
Chicken with black-bean sauce and rice – 413 Calories
Lasagne – 428 Calories
Lamb dopiaza – 285 Calories (Add 100 g (3^1/2 oz) boiled rice)

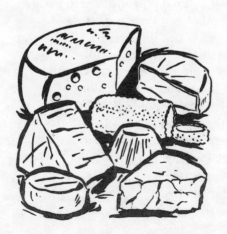

7-Day 1,500 Calorie Slimming Plan

Although weight loss is slower on a 1,500 Calorie diet, for some people it is more socially acceptable and therefore a more successful way of dieting than the 1,200 Calorie diet. The diet follows the same principles as the 1,200 Calorie diet, but allows more fruit and bread or cereals, plus an extra treat.

Daily allowance
300 ml (1/2 pt) skimmed milk or semi-skimmed milk
    or 150 ml (1/4 pint) skimmed milk and 100 ml
    (4 fl oz) low-fat natural yogurt
    or 200 ml (7 fl oz) soya milk
25 g (1 oz) low-fat spread
    or 15 g (1/2 oz) polyunsaturated margarine
    or 20 ml (4 tsp) French dressing
    or 10 ml (2 tsp) unsaturated oil
A portion of fresh fruit.

Plus *an extra item each day:*
1 small glass of white or red wine
300 ml (1/2 pint) of lager or beer
150 ml (1/4 pint) of orange juice
1 extra slice of bread
1 digestive biscuit
1 low-fat fruit yogurt
A portion of fruit.

BREAKFAST

Monday
1 glass fresh orange juice
1 large, thick slice wholemeal toast
scraping of polyunsaturated margarine
10 ml (2 tsp) marmalade or jam or lemon curd
45 ml (3 tbsp) bran flakes

Tuesday
$1/2$ grapefruit
45 ml (3 large tbsp) bran flakes
milk from allowance
1 large, thick slice Granary bread
scraping of polyunsaturated margarine
10 ml (2 tsp) marmalade or jam or lemon curd

Wednesday
1 apple sliced and mixed with 45 ml (3 large tbsp)
unsweetened muesli
milk from allowance
1 large, thick slice wholemeal bread
scraping of polyunsaturated margarine
10 ml (2 tsp) marmalade or jam or lemon curd

Thursday
1 glass fresh orange juice
2 wholewheat biscuits
milk from allowance

——————————— *Friday* ———————————
1 banana, sliced and mixed with
45 ml (3 large tbsp) bran flakes
milk from allowance
1 large, thick slice wholemeal bread
scraping of polyunsaturated margarine
10 ml (2 tsp) marmalade or jam
or lemon curd

——————————— *Saturday* ———————————
1 glass fresh orange juice
1 large, thick slice Granary bread
1 small slice lean ham or 1 small cheese triangle
45 ml (3 tbsp) bran flakes
milk from allowance

——————————— *Sunday* ———————————
$1/2$ grapefruit
2 large, thick slices wholemeal toast
Mushrooms cooked with 7 g ($1/4$ oz) polyunsaturated
fat spread in non-stick pan
2 small rashers of lean back bacon, grilled
Vegetarian option: 1 poached egg

LUNCH

——————————— *Monday* ———————————
50 g (2 oz) lean roast chicken meat and
Italian Salad (p.173) sandwich made with
2 large, thick slices wholemeal bread
1 apple

Vegetarian option: 1 hard-boiled egg, sliced and
Italian Salad (p.173) sandwich made with
2 large, thick slices wholemeal bread
1 apple

--- *Tuesday* ---

225 g (8 oz) jacket potato filled with
150 g (5 oz) baked beans and
50 g (2 oz) lean ham and chopped tomato salad
1 banana

Vegetarian option: 225 g (8 oz) jacket potato
filled with 150 g (5 oz) baked beans
and 15 g ($^{1}/_{2}$ oz) Parmesan cheese and
chopped tomato salad
1 banana

--- *Wednesday* ---

Mexican Tuna (p.122) salad sandwich made with
2 large, thick slices Granary bread and
an extra tomato
1 orange

Vegetarian option: 50 g (2 oz) Hummus (p.153)
salad sandwich made with
2 large, thick slices of Granary bread
1 orange

--- *Thursday* ---

50 g (2 oz) reduced-fat hard cheese and salad
sandwich made from a large brown bap
1 pear
1 low-fat fruit yogurt

————————————— *Friday* —————————————
175 g (6 oz) jacket potato with
75 g (3 oz) cottage cheese, grated carrots and
15 g ($^1/_2$ oz) nuts
1 portion fresh fruit salad

————————————— *Saturday* —————————————
Black Bean Soup (p.153)
ham and salad sandwich made with
2 large, thick slices of wholemeal bread and
50 g (2 oz) lean ham
1 apple
Vegetarian option: Black Bean Soup (p.153)
pitta bread filled with salad and
50 g (2 oz) grated Edam cheese
1 apple

————————————— *Sunday* —————————————
90 g (3$^1/_2$ oz) lean roast leg of lamb
Ratatouille (p.130)
peas
150 g (5 oz) cooked basmati rice
Fruit Kebabs (p.193)
Vegetarian option: 50 g (2 oz) reduced-fat
hard cheese
150 g (5 oz) cooked basmati rice
Ratatouille (p.130)
peas
Fruit Kebabs (p.193)

EVENING

Monday
Butterbean and Mushroom Bake (p.151)
grated carrot salad
tomato salad
200 g (7 oz) jacket potato
1 glass fresh orange juice
1 low-fat fruit yogurt

Tuesday
Chicken with Watercress Sauce (p.172)
150 g (5 oz) cooked pasta
broccoli
carrots
Pears with Fresh Ginger (p.189)
Vegetarian option: 1 large Stuffed Pepper (p.162)
broccoli
carrots
1 bread roll
Pears with Ginger (p.189)

Wednesday
100 g (3^1/$_2$ oz) fish or chicken tikka kebab
made with 100 g (3^1/$_2$ oz)
Yogurt Tandoori Marinade (p.196)
150 g (5 oz) cooked Spicy Rice (p.131)
Turkish Salad (p.174)
lettuce
fresh mango and 1 scoop Raspberry Sorbet (p.183)
Vegetarian option: 225 g (8 oz) Vegetable
Chilli (p.155)
150 g (5 oz) cooked Spicy Rice (p.131)

Turkish Salad (p.174)
lettuce
fresh mango and 1 scoop Raspberry Sorbet (p.183)

––––––––––––––––– *Thursday* –––––––––––––––––
Pasta with Aubergine and Tomato Sauce (p.144)
mixed salad
Winter Salad (p.175)
fresh fruit salad

––––––––––––––––– *Friday* –––––––––––––––––
150 g (5 oz) boiled rice
Stir-fry Vegetables (p.160) with 75 g (3 oz) pork
baked apple with raisins
low-fat yogurt from allowance
Vegetarian option: Stir-fry Vegetables (p.160)
with 25 g (1 oz) flaked toasted almonds
150 g (5 oz) boiled rice
baked apple and raisins and low-fat yogurt
from allowance

––––––––––––––––– *Saturday* –––––––––––––––––
200 g (7 oz) boiled new potatoes
Green beans in Tomato Sauce (p.168)
100 g (3^1/2 oz) baked salmon
Peach Brûlée (p.188)
Vegetarian option: Spinach and
Cheese Squares (p.165)
200 g (7 oz) boiled new potatoes
Green beans in Tomato Sauce (p.168)
Peach Brûlée (p.188)

Sunday
75 g (3 oz) Bean Pâté (p.156)
2 pitta bread with green salad
grapes

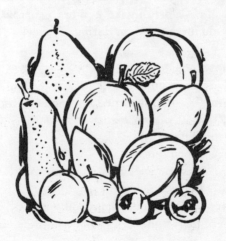

Everyday 7-Day 2,000 Calorie Eating Plan

This diet has been developed to show how you could adapt the 28-Day Slimming Plan (which is 1,200 Calories per day) once you have stopped dieting, or for another member of your family who is not on a diet. Most of us eat and drink more when we are at home, so the Calorie intake is more generous at the weekend and more stringent during the week.

Daily allowance
300 ml (¹/₂ pint) skimmed or semi-skimmed milk
   or 150 ml (¹/₄ pint) skimmed milk and 100 ml
   (4 fl oz) low-fat natural yogurt
   or 200 ml (7 fl oz) soya milk.
25 g (1 oz) low-fat spread
   or 15 g (¹/₂ oz) polyunsaturated margarine
   or 20 ml (4 tsp) French dressing
   or 10 ml (2 tsp) polyunsaturated oil
A portion of fresh fruit.

BREAKFAST

Monday

1 glass fresh orange juice
1 large, thick slice wholemeal toast
scraping of polyunsaturated margarine
10 ml (2 tsp) marmalade or jam
or lemon curd
45 ml (3 tbsp) bran flakes, milk from allowance

Tuesday

$1/2$ grapefruit
45 ml (3 tbsp) bran flakes, milk from allowance
1 large, thick slice Granary bread
scraping of polyunsaturated margarine
10 ml (2 tsp) marmalade or jam
or lemon curd

Wednesday

1 apple sliced and mixed with 45 ml (3 tbsp)
unsweetened museli, milk from allowance
1 large, thick slice wholemeal bread
scraping of polyunsaturated margarine
10 ml (2 tsp) marmalade or jam
or lemon curd

Thursday

1 glass fresh orange juice
1 wholemeal muffin
scraping of polyunsaturated margarine
yeast extract
2 Weetabix, milk from allowance

Friday

1 banana, sliced and mixed with
45 ml (3 tbsp) bran flakes
milk from allowance
1 large, thick slice wholemeal bread
scraping of polyunsaturated margarine
10 ml (2 tsp) marmalade or jam
or lemon curd

Saturday

1 glass fresh orange juice
1 large, thick slice Granary bread
1 small slice lean ham or
1 small cheese triangle
45 ml (3 tbsp) bran flakes
milk from allowance

Sunday

$1/2$ grapefruit
2 large, thick slices wholemeal toast
mushrooms cooked with 7 g ($1/4$ oz)
polyunsaturated spread in non-stick pan
2 small rashers lean back bacon, grilled
Vegetarian option: 1 poached egg

LUNCHES

Monday

50 g (2 oz) lean roast chicken meat and
Italian Salad (p.173) sandwich made with
2 large, thick slices wholemeal bread
1 apple
Vegetarian option: 1 hard-boiled egg, sliced and
Italian Salad (p.173) sandwich made with
2 large, thick slices wholemeal bread
1 apple

Tuesday

225 g (8 oz) jacket potato filled with
150 g (5 oz) baked beans and 50 g (2 oz) lean ham
and chopped tomato salad
1 banana
Vegetarian option: 225 g (8 oz) jacket potato filled
with 150 g (5 oz) baked beans and 15 g ($^1/2$ oz)
Parmesan cheese and
chopped tomato salad
1 banana

Wednesday

Mexican Tuna (p.122) salad sandwich made with
2 large, thick slices Granary bread
and an extra tomato
1 orange
Vegetarian option: 50 g (2 oz) Hummus (p.153)
salad sandwich made with 2 large,
thick slices Granary bread
1 orange

Thursday

50 g (2 oz) reduced-fat hard cheese and salad
sandwich made from a large brown bap
1 pear
1 low-fat fruit yogurt

Friday

175 g (6 oz) jacket potato with
75 g (3 oz) cottage cheese, grated carrot and
15 g (^{1}/2 oz) nuts
1 portion fresh fruit salad

Saturday

Black Bean Soup (p.153)
ham and salad sandwich made with
2 large, thick slices wholemeal bread
and 50 g (2 oz) lean ham
1 apple
Vegetarian option: Black Bean Soup (p.153)
pitta bread filled with salad and
50 g (2 oz) grated Edam cheese
1 apple

Sunday

100 g (3^1/2 oz) lean roast leg of lamb
Ratatouille (p.130)
peas
200 g (7 oz) cooked basmati rice
Fruit Kebabs (p.193)

Vegetarian option: 50 g (2 oz) reduced-fat
hard cheese
200 g (7 oz) cooked basmati rice
Ratatouille (p.130)
peas
Fruit Kebabs (p.193)

MID-AFTERNOON SNACKS

Tuesday

2 digestive biscuits

Thursday

1 sultana scone with scraping of butter

Saturday

1 large slice chocolate cake with butter-cream icing

EVENING

Monday

Butterbean and Mushroom Bake (p.151)
grated carrot salad
tomato salad
225 g (8 oz) jacket potato
1 glass fresh orange juice
1 low-fat fruit yogurt

———————————— *Tuesday* ————————————

Chicken with Watercress Sauce (p.172)
200 g (7 oz) cooked pasta
broccoli
carrots
Pears with Fresh Ginger (p.189)
2 glasses dry white wine
Vegetarian option: 1 large Stuffed Pepper (p.162)
broccoli, carrots
1 bread roll
Pears with Fresh Ginger (p.189)
2 glasses dry white wine

———————————— *Wednesday* ————————————

100 g (3^1/2 oz) fish or chicken tikka kebab made
with 100 g (3^1/2 oz) Yogurt Tandoori
Marinade (p.196)
150 g (5 oz) oven chips
Turkish Salad (p.174)
lettuce
fresh mango and 1 scoop Raspberry Sorbet (p.183)
Vegetarian option: 225 g (8 oz) Vegetable
Chilli (p.155)
200 g (7 oz) cooked Spicy Rice (p.131)
Turkish Salad (p.174)
lettuce
fresh mango and 1 scoop Raspberry Sorbet (p.183)

———————————— *Thursday* ————————————

Pasta with Aubergine and Tomato Sauce (p.144)
mixed salad, Winter Salad (p.175)
2 scoops Lemon Sorbet (p.183)
2 glasses red wine

Friday

200 g (7 oz) boiled rice
Stir-fry Vegetables (p.160) with 75 g (3 oz) pork
baked apple with raisins and
low-fat yogurt from allowance
1 small glass of lager
Vegetarian option: Stir-fry Vegetables (p.160)
with 25 g (1 oz) flaked toasted almonds
200 g (7 oz) boiled rice
baked apple and raisins and
low-fat yogurt from allowance
1 small glass of lager

Saturday

225 g (8 oz) boiled new potatoes
Green Beans in Tomato Sauce (p.168)
100 g (3$^{1}/_{2}$ oz) baked salmon
Peach Brûlée (p.188)
2 glasses dry white wine
Vegetarian option: Spinach and
Cheese Squares (p.165)
225 g (8 oz) boiled new potatoes
Green Beans in Tomato Sauce (p.168)
Peach Brûlée (p.188)
2 glasses dry white wine

Sunday

75 g (3 oz) Bean Pâté (p.156)
2 pitta bread with green salad
grapes
50 g (2 oz) milk chocolate

A Diet You Can Share

The *Eat for Life* plans cater for you, your family and even your friends. If you follow the suggestions and helpful, at-a-glance menus you can entertain at home with everything from barbecues to Sunday lunch and enjoy eating out in restaurants as well.

~ *Menus for entertaining* ~

Vegetarian Meal

Vegetable Curry (p.163)
Basmati rice (boiled)
Dhal (p.149)
Raita (p.201)
Sliced tomatoes
Pappads

Dried Fruit Salad (p.189) with
Almond Biscuits (p.184)

Barbecue

Mushroom à la Grecque (p.159)
Pitta bread
Mexican Beans and Rice (p.138)
West Indian Pork (p.210)
Mango and Tomato Salsa (p.203)
Carrot and Nut Salad (p.176)
Garden Salad (p.176)

Sliced tomatoes
Fresh Fruit Platter (p.186) with
Raspberry Sauce (p.195)

―――――――― **Dinner Party 1** ――――――――

Tom Yam Gung (Thai fish soup) (p.208)

Venison Ragout (p.209)
Green Beans with Almonds (p.165)
Mixed steamed vegetables
(Mange tout, carrots, baby sweetcorn)
Boiled new potatoes

Simple Trifle (p.191)

―――――――― **Dinner Party 2** ――――――――

Bruschetta (p.126)

Seafood Risotto (p.133)
Large mixed salad (lettuce, tomatoes, radish,
cucumber, carrots)

Peaches Stuffed with Almonds (p.190)

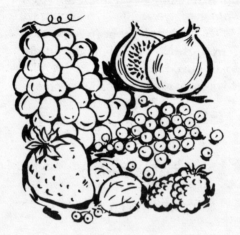

PART THREE
Eat for Life Recipes

Use these recipes to help you adopt the *Eat for Life* approach to slimming and healthy eating. The recipes are grouped according to starchy foods, on which you should base your meal. Slimmers use these recipes with the 28-day and the 7-day Slimming Plans as well as the Easy Option Slimming Plan. They also fit into the Everyday Eating Plan and can be used for entertaining.

~ Putting Eat for Life Rules
into your own recipes ~

- Swap lard, dripping, butter and ghee for low-fat spreads, or vegetable oils or margarines that are high in polyunsaturates or low-fat spreads.
- Use the minimum amount of fat in recipes and when cooking. Keep frying to a minimum; instead bake, steam, boil, poach, grill, dry roast or microwave.
- Don't have too many pastry and pie dishes.
- Swap full-fat milk in recipes for skimmed milk.
- Replace cream, cream cheese and other full-fat soft cheeses with fromage frais or other low-fat soft cheeses and different types of yogurt.
- Flavour cottage cheese or other low-fat cheeses with garlic and herbs instead of using standard full-fat flavoured creamy cheeses.
- Use only a little hard cheese, because it is very high in fat. Full-flavoured mature Cheddar-style

COOKING FAT PROFILES

	Saturated g/100g	Mono-unsaturated g/100g	Polyun-saturated g/100g
Beef dripping	43	48	4
Butter	49	26	2
Coconut oil	85	7	2
Corn oil	17	29	49
Lard	42	42	9
Olive oil	14	70	11
Peanut oil	45	42	8
Polyunsaturated margarine	19	16	60
Safflower seed oil	19	48	28
Soyabean oil	10	13	72
Sunflower seed oil	14	24	57

makes a little go a long way. Other tasty cheeses that have a lot of flavour are Gruyère, Emmenthal, Parmesan.

- Cut off all visible fat on meat and use only lean meat. Don't use sausagemeat, luncheon meats, fatty salamis, sausages, meat pies, pâtés, standard mince – or use them only rarely.

- If you make soups, casseroles, stocks etc, skim off any fat before serving. Preferably make them the day before to allow them to become completely cold for thorough fat removal.

- Cut down on the amount of salt in cooking and recipes. Spices, herbs and lemon and lime juice give flavour.

- Stock cubes are very salty. Make your own stock, or use low-salt stock cubes.
- Go easy on the soy sauce, barbecue sauce and other high salt sauces.
- In general, cut down on fatty sauces with food. Instead of gravy made with fat from the joint, serve meat with the juices from the meat or a little stock.
- Don't make regular use of creamed and desiccated coconut – it is very high in saturated fat.

FATS IN MEAT		
PERCENTAGE FATTY ACIDS		
Saturated	Mono-unsaturated	Polyun-saturated
Beef, sirloin, for roasting		
45	49	4
Lamb, leg, for roasting		
52	41	5
Pork, leg, for roasting		
43	48	8
Chicken, roast, meat and skin		
35	48	15
Turkey, roast, meat only		
37	27	30
Bacon, back, grilled		
43	48	8
Liver, lamb's, fried		
42	35	18

~ *Three steps to healthier cooking and eating* ~

Step 1
- Grill food whenever possible.
- Replace white or brown bread with wholemeal as your principal type of bread.
- Cut out sugar in drinks.
- Choose fruit juice or water instead of sugary drinks.
- Use skimmed or semi-skimmed milk instead of whole milk, and yogurt instead of cream.
- Use oils and spreads rich in polyunsaturates.
- Choose lean meat, poultry and fish.

Step 2
- Start to cut down on the overall amount of fat you use in cooking. Replace rice, pasta and breakfast cereals with wholemeal varieties.
- Cut down on between-meal sugary snacks like cakes, biscuits, sweets and chocolates. Snack instead on bread, and fruit.
- Increase the amount of fruit and vegetables you eat, aiming for five portions of fruit, vegetables or salad a day.

Step 3
- Eat more beans and pulses such as lentils, beans, chick peas.
- Cut down on the amount of fatty meat you eat, particularly processed meats such as sausages, hamburgers, pâté.

- Make sure the portions of meat and fish you eat are not too large.
- Cut down on the amount of fatty cheeses you eat.
- Try to reduce the amount of salt added during cooking and at the table.
- Try to keep within the recommended limit (see pages 31–2) when drinking alcohol.

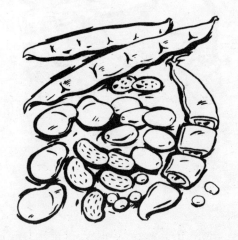

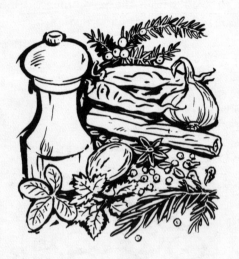

~ *The recipes* ~

SANDWICHES AND FILLINGS

—

MEXICAN TUNA FILLING

SERVES 2

175 g (6 oz) canned tuna fish • $^1/_4$ green pepper, deseeded and chopped

50 g (2 oz) cooked sweetcorn • 100 g ($3^1/_2$ oz) cooked kidney beans

dash of Tabasco sauce (optional)

Mix tuna, pepper, sweetcorn, kidney beans and Tabasco
sauce together in a bowl.

> *167 Kcal/701 KJ • 26.8 g Protein • 9.2 g Carbohydrate of which: sugars 2.9 g •*
> *2.7 g Fat of which: saturates 0.1 g • 0.2 g Sodium • 1.7 g Dietary Fibre*

—

SMOKED MACKEREL PÂTÉ

SERVES 2

100 g ($3^1/_2$ oz) smoked mackerel • 50 g (2 oz) low-fat curd cheese

$^1/_2$ lemon – squeezed

Remove the skin and bones from the smoked mackerel.
Place in a liquidiser with cheese and lemon.

> *149 Kcal/621 KJ • 15.1 g Protein • 1.1 g Carbohydrate of which: sugars 1.1 g •*
> *9.3 g Fat of which: saturates 3.4 g • 0.5 g Sodium • no Dietary Fibre*

●

EGG AND WATERCRESS FILLING

SERVES 1

1 egg, hard boiled • 25 g (1 oz) watercress, finely chopped

2 tsp (10 ml) low-calorie mayonaise

Chop the hard-boiled egg and mix with the watercress and mayonnaise.

125 Kcal/522 KJ • 9.2 g Protein • 1.2 g Carbohydrate of which: 0.8 sugars • 9.4 g Fat of which: 1.9 g saturates • 0.2 g Sodium • 1.7 g Dietary Fibre

●

NIÇOISE FILLING

SERVES 2

1 egg, hard boiled • 75 g (3 oz) canned tuna fish

5 slices red pepper, chopped • 3 black olives, chopped

2 tsp (10 ml) low-calorie mayonaise • 1/2 tsp wine vinegar

Chop the hard-boiled egg and mix with the tuna, pepper, olives, mayonnaise and vinegar in a bowl.

124 Kcal/516 KJ • 14.5 g Protein • 1.0 g Carbohydrate of which: sugars 0.7 g • 6.9 g Fat of which: saturates 1.2 g • 0.8 g Sodium • 0.9 Dietary Fibre

●

PRAWN AND CABBAGE FILLING

SERVES 2

100 g (3¹/₂ oz) prawns • 100 g (3¹/₂ oz) white cabbage, finely shredded

15 ml (1 tbsp) lemon juice • 10 ml (2 tsp) low-calorie mayonnaise

Mix together prawns, cabbage, lemon juice and mayonnaise.

80 Kcal/334 KJ • 12.4 g Protein • 2.5 g Carbohydrate of which: sugars 2.3 g •
2.3 g Fat of which: saturates 0.1 g • 0.9 g Sodium • 1.4 g Dietary Fibre

●

CHICKEN AND BLUE CHEESE SALAD TOASTED SANDWICH

SERVES 2

75 g (3 oz) roasted chicken • 50 g (2 oz) dolcelatte, grated

4 large thick slices wholemeal bread • 10 ml (2 tsp) low-fat spread

1 sliced tomato • lettuce

Thinly slice the chicken. Toast the bread and spread with the low-fat spread. Place the salad, cheese and chicken mixture evenly between the bread.

182 Kcal/763 KJ • 12.1 g Protein • 17.1 g Carbohydrate of which: sugars 1.9 g •
7.7 g Fat of which: saturates 3.8 g • 0.3 g Sodium • 2.5 g Dietary Fibre

●

TABOULLEH

SERVES 2

| 50 g (2 oz) bulghur or cracked wheat • large chuck of cucumber |
| 1/3 green pepper deseeded and finely diced • small red onion, diced |
| 30ml (2 tbsp) freshly chopped mint • juice of 1/2 lemon • black pepper |

Cook the wheat in twice its volume of boiling water for 10 minutes, or leave it to stand in the same amount of just boiled water for 15 minutes until the grain has swelled and softened. Drain and squeeze out moisture and place the wheat in a bowl. Stir in the remaining ingredients.

103 Kcal/431 KJ • 3.2 g Protein • 22g Carbohydrate of which: sugar 2.8 g • 0.6 Fat of which: saturates trace • trace Sodium • 0.7 g Dietary Fibre

●

CHICKEN AND TABOULLEH SANDWICH

SERVES 1

| 2 slices wholemeal bread • 7 g (1/4 oz) low-fat spread |
| 50 g (2 oz) lean roast chicken • 30 ml (2 tbsp) taboulleh (see above) |

Thinly spread the bread with the spread. Place chicken and taboulleh on one slice of bread, top with the second slice.

373 Kcal/1574 KJ • 24.2 g Protein • 54.8 g Carbohydrate, of which: 3.3 g sugars • 7.8 g Fat of which: 1.5 g saturates • 0.7 g Sodium • 6.8 g Dietary Fibre

CRAB STUFFED PITTA BREAD

SERVES 1

60 g (2¹/₂ oz) white crab meat • 50 g (2 oz) white cabbage, finely chopped
5 ml (1 tsp) lemon juice • 5 ml (1 tsp) low-calorie mayonnaise
1 large wholemeal pitta bread

Mix the cabbage, lemon juice and mayonnaise together in a bowl. Put the mixture inside the pitta bread, then top with the crab meat.

390 Kcal/1645 KJ • 22.0 g Protein • 57.0 g Carbohydrate, of which: 4.2 g sugars • 9.9 g Fat, of which: 1.2 g saturates • 0.7 g Sodium • 9.9 g Dietary Fibre

BRUSCHETTA

SERVES 2

8 cherry tomatoes, cut in half
2 thick slices ciabatta bread
2 tbsp (30 ml) black olive pâté
freshly chopped basil

Grill the tomatoes under a hot grill. At the same time toast the bread and spread one side with the olive paste. Top with the tomatoes and basil.

170 Kcal/709 KJ • 5.6 g Protein • 26.4 g Carbohydrates, of which: sugars 3.7 g 5.4 g Fat of which: saturates 0.8 g • 0.7 g Sodium • 4.6 g Dietary Fibre

POTATOES

SUMMER SOUP

SERVES 4

750 ml (1¹/₄ pints) chicken or vegetable stock

350 g (12 oz) potatoes, scrubbed and cut into large pieces

1 large onion, peeled and chopped • 2 leeks, well rinsed and sliced

10 ml (2 tsp) olive oil • 50 g (2 oz) basil leaves, chopped

100 g (3¹/₂ oz) watercress • ground black pepper

Combine the stock, potatoes and onion in a large saucepan. Cook until the potatoes are tender (about 20 minutes). Heat oil in a non-stick fry pan and sauté leeks for 10 minutes until almost tender. Add the basil and watercress and cook for a further 5 minutes. Purée the soup in the blender. Add black pepper. Return to the pan and heat gently.

137 Kcal/572 KJ • 5.1 g Protein • 24.9 g Carbohydrate, of which: 6.9 g sugars • 2.7 g Fat, of which: 0.4 g saturates • 0.2 g Sodium • 6.4 g Dietary Fibre

INDIAN POTATOES

SERVES 4

450 g (1 lb) potatoes, scrubbed and chopped into small pieces

1 cauliflower, chopped into small florets • 10 ml (2 tsp) oil

5 ml (1 tsp) turmeric • 2.5 ml (1/2 tsp) cumin seeds

ground black pepper • 100 g (3 1/2 oz) mushrooms

Par-boil the potatoes for 5 minutes, then add the cauliflower and cook for a further 4 minutes. Drain. Heat oil in a wok and then add the spices. Cook for about 1 minute and then add the vegetables. Cook for 5 minutes or until the vegetables are tender.

128 Kcal (534 Kj) • 3.9 g Protein • 23.4 g Carbohydrate, of which: 1.4 g sugars • 2.8 g Fat, of which: 0.4 g saturates • trace Sodium • 3.8 g Dietary Fibre

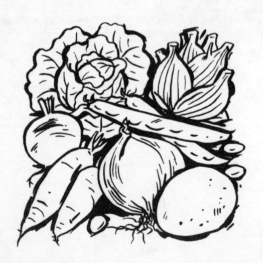

TUNA AND POTATO BAKE

SERVES 4

350 g (12 oz) onion, peeled and sliced • 1 clove garlic, crushed
5 ml (1 tsp) sunflower oil • 400 g (14 oz) chopped canned tomatoes
15 ml (1 tbsp) tomato purée • 200 g (7 oz) canned tuna, drained
12 black olives, chopped • pinch mixed herbs
2.5 ml (1/2 tsp) sugar • 350 g (12 oz) potatoes, scrubbed and cooked
25 g (1 oz) breadcrumbs

Soften onion and garlic in oil in a non-stick fry pan. Add
tomatoes and tomato purée and simmer for about 10
minutes. Add tuna, black olives, herbs and sugar and cook for
a further 5 minutes. Meanwhile heat the oven to 190°C,
375°F mark 5. Grease an ovenproof dish and add potatoes
and sauce ending with a layer of sauce. Sprinkle with
breadcrumbs and cook for 40 minutes.

*217 Kcal/908 KJ • 18.2 g Protein • 30.7 g Carbohydrate, of which: 8.8 g sugars •
3.2 g Fat, of which: 0.4 g saturates • 0.2 g sodium • 5.3 g Dietary Fibre*

HUNGARIAN POTATOES

SERVES 4

10 ml (2 tsp) olive oil • 1 large onion, peeled and chopped
2 cloves garlic, crushed • 1 large aubergine, diced
2 red peppers, deseeded and sliced • 15 ml (1 tbsp) paprika
100 g (4 oz) mushrooms, sliced • 400 g (14 oz) chopped canned tomatoes
45 ml (3 tbsp) tomato purée • sprig of thyme
350 g (12 oz) potatoes, scrubbed and cooked until just tender
ground black pepper • 30 ml (2 tbsp) water

Heat oil in a large casserole dish. Add the onion and cook over a low heat for 10 minutes or until brown. Add garlic and cook for a further 2 minutes. Add the aubergine and pepper, cover with a lid and cook for a further 5 minutes. Add the paprika and cook for 2 minutes. Mix in the remaining vegetables, tomato purée, thyme and 2 tablespoons water and simmer for 45 – 60 minutes or until cooked.

159 Kcal/667 KJ • 5.6 g Protein • 3.2 g Carbohydrate of which: sugars 0.4 g • 29.1 g Fat of which: saturates 10.8 g • trace Sodium • 6.3 g Dietary Fibre

Variations: Chick Pea Hot Pot. Delete the potatoes from the above recipe and add 400 g (14 oz) cooked chick peas instead. Add 5 ml (1 tsp) ground cinnamon as well as the other seasoning.

184 Kcal/771 KJ • 11.4 g Protein • 3.5 g Fat of which: saturates 0.4 g • 29 g Carbohydrate of which: sugars 11.9 g • trace Sodium • 10.5 g Dietary Fibre

Ratatouille. Delete the potatoes and mushrooms from the above recipe and add 1 lb (450 g) sliced courgettes at the same time as the aubergine. Delete the paprika.

117 Kcal/492 KJ • 6.1 g Protein • 3.6 g Fat of which: saturates 0.4 g • 17.0 g Carbohydrate of which: sugars 10.4 g • trace Sodium • 5.5 g Dietary Fibre

RICE

●

ARROZ VERDE

SERVES 4

5 ml (1 tsp) sunflower oil • 2 green peppers, deseeded and chopped

¹/₂ onion, peeled and finely chopped

1 green chilli, deseeded and finely chopped or
pinch chilli powder • 60 ml (4 tbsp) chopped fresh parsley

225 g (8 oz) long grain white rice • 600 ml (1 pint) vegetable stock

ground black pepper

Heat the oil in a large saucepan and fry the peppers, onion
and chilli for 5 minutes. Add the remaining ingredients, bring
to the boil, cover and simmer for 12 minutes or until the rice
is tender.

*240 Kcal/1005 KJ • 5.8 g Protein • 48.2 g Carbohydrate, of which: 3.1 g sugars •
2.4 g Fat, of which: 0.3 g saturates • 0.2 g Sodium • 1.0 g Dietary Fibre*

●

SPICY RICE

SERVES 4

225 g (8 oz) long grain brown rice • 5 ml (1 tsp) ground turmeric

1 stick cinnamon • 1 bay leaf

4 green cardamon pods • 6 black peppercorns

Put all the ingredients in a saucepan with enough water and
bring to the boil. Cook for 35 minutes or until the rice is
tender. Drain and serve.

*205 Kcal/872 KJ • 3.9 g Protein • 46.5 g Carbohydrate, of which: 0.7 g sugars •
1.7 g Fat, of which: no saturates trace Sodium • 2.1 g Dietary Fibre*

●

NASI GORENG (WITH CHICKEN OR EGG)

SERVES 4

10 ml (2 tsp) sunflower oil • 4 small chicken breasts
2 large onions, peeled and chopped • 3 cloves garlic, crushed
1.25 ml (1/4 tsp) chilli powder • 1.25 ml (1/4 tsp) laos (optional)
10 ml (2 tsp) ground cumin • 5 ml (1 tsp) ground coriander
30 ml (2 tbsp) soy sauce • 15 ml (1 tbsp) tomato ketchup
275 g (10 oz) long grain brown rice, cooked

Heat the oil in a large non-stick pan and cook the chicken breasts for about 15 – 20 minutes. Remove the chicken and allow to cool. Add the onions to the pan and cook for 15 minutes until well browned. Add the garlic and cook for a further 1 minute. Stir in the spices and cook for 2 minutes. Cut the chicken breasts into small pieces and add to the pan with the soy sauce, tomato ketchup and brown rice. Cover and cook for 20 minutes, stirring frequently. Add 15 – 30 ml (1 – 2 tbsp) water if necessary.

267 Kcal/1117 KJ • 24.9 g Protein • 28.3 g Carbohydrate, of which: 4.7 g sugars • 6.7 g Fat, of which: 1.4 g saturates • 0.1 g Sodium • 1.8 g Dietary Fibre

Variation: Egg Nasi Goreng. Instead of using chicken, make the Nasi Goreng with an omelette. Make a flat omelette with 4 eggs. When cooked, cut into strips and add 5 minutes before serving. If all the family aren't vegetarian, separate the dish into the appropriate portions after cooking the spices. Add the chicken to the portion for meat eaters and later add the omelette to the other portion.

265 Kcal/1109 KJ • 9.6 g Protein • 28.3 g Carbohydrate, of which: 4.7 g sugars • 13.4 g Fat, of which: 4.8 g saturates • 0.7 g Sodium • 1.8 g Dietary Fibre

SEAFOOD RISOTTO

SERVES 4

10 ml (2 tsp) sunflower oil • 1 large onion, peeled and chopped

2 cloves garlic, crushed • 275 g (10 oz) American long grain rice

150 ml (1/4 pint) dry white wine • 450 ml (3/4 pint) vegetable stock

150 g (5 oz) prepared squid, chopped • 225 g (8 oz) peeled prawns

1 red pepper, deseeded and chopped • 1 large courgette, sliced

1 large pinch chilli powder

90 ml (6 tbsp) chopped fresh mixed herbs
such as basil, coriander and parsley

Heat the oil in a large heavy casserole and slowly cook the onion for 10 minutes. Add the garlic and rice and cook for a further 4 minutes. Add the wine and simmer until most of the liquid is absorbed. Stir in half of the stock and simmer until the liquid is absorbed, stirring frequently. Add the remainder of the stock and simmer until the liquid is absorbed. Mix in the fish, cover and cook for 5 minutes. Stir in the vegetables and chilli powder, cover and cook for a further 7 minutes. Add more water if the risotto starts to dry out. Finally add the herbs, stir and then serve.

389 Kcal/1647 KJ • 16.3 g Protein • 65.5 g Carbohydrate, of which: 5.1 g sugars • 6.2 g Fat, of which: 0.4 g saturates • 0.4 g Sodium • 3.2 g Dietary Fibre

●

BROWN RICE SALAD

SERVES 4

225 g (8 oz) long grain brown rice, cooked

150 g (5 oz) French beans, trimmed • 75 g (3 oz) sweetcorn, cooked

1/2 red pepper, deseeded and chopped • 75 g (3 oz) seedless grapes

3 spring onions, chopped

350 g (12 oz) cooked chicken, cubed (optional)

30 ml (2 tbsp) French Dressing (see page 205)

Mix all the ingredients together in a large bowl.

412 Kcal/1736 KJ • 27.1 g Protein • 52.8 g Carbohydrate, of which: 5.5 g sugars
• 11.2 g Fat, of which: 2.3 g saturates • 0.2 g Sodium • 4.6 g Dietary Fibre

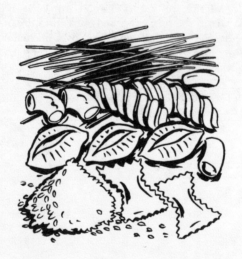

LEEK OR COURGETTE RISOTTO

SERVES 4

10 ml (2 tsp) sunflower oil • 1 small onion, peeled and sliced
1 clove garlic, crushed • 275 g (10 oz) leeks, washed and sliced, or 350 g (12 oz) courgettes, sliced
350 g (12 oz) risotto rice • 1.5 litres (2½ pints) vegetable stock
large handful parsley, chopped
15 ml (1 tbsp) grated Parmesan cheese

Heat the oil in a large saucepan and cook the onion and garlic until soft, about 5 minutes. Add the leeks or courgettes and cook for 7 minutes, stirring frequently. Add the rice and stir a couple of times until it is coated with oil. Stir in the stock, a ladleful at a time, always waiting for the previous addition to be absorbed before adding the next ladleful. Cook the rice for about 20 minutes or until al dente. As soon as the rice is tender, stir in the parsley and Parmesan cheese and serve.

278 Kcal/1159 KJ • 7.4 g Protein • 29.5 g Carbohydrate, of which: 11.0 g sugars • 14.7 g Fat, of which: 1.6 g saturates • 0.4 g Sodium • 4.4 g Dietary Fibre

●

LEMON RICE
WITH CASHEWS

SERVES 4

225 g (8 oz) easy cook brown rice • 15 ml (1 tbsp) grated lemon rind

juice of 1 lemon • 50 g (2 oz) cashew nuts (not for dieters!)

ground black pepper

Cook the rice in a pan of boiling water until tender, then drain. Add the remaining ingredients and stir over a low heat for 3 minutes for flavours to mix. Serve.

WITHOUT CASHEWS
204 Kcal/867 KJ • 3.9 g Protein • 46.4 g Carbohydrate, of which: 1.4 g sugars •
1.6 g Fat, of which: no saturates • trace Sodium • 3.2 g Dietary Fibre

---

WITH CASHEWS
274 Kcal/1160 KJ • 6.1 g Protein • 49.9 g Carbohydrate, of which: 1.4 g sugars •
7.3 g Fat, of which: no saturates • trace Sodium • 3.2 g Dietary Fibre

---

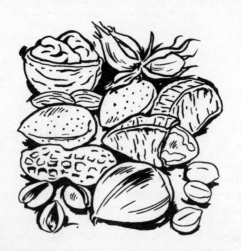

●

KEDGEREE

SERVES 4

225 g (8 oz) easy cook brown rice • 600 ml (1 pint) fish stock

225 g (8 oz) mange tout • 400 g (14 oz) salmon

1 bay leaf • 6 whole black peppercorns

juice of 1 lemon • ground black pepper

large handful parsley, chopped • 2 spring onions, chopped

Cook the rice in the stock. When nearly cooked, add the mange tout and cook for a further 5 minutes. Drain. Meanwhile, place the fish in a frying pan with the bay leaf, peppercorns and the juice from $1/2$ the lemon. Add just enough water to cover the fish and simmer for 15 minutes or until tender. Drain and flake the fish into large chunks, discarding any bones. Mix together the rice, fish, black pepper, remaining lemon juice, parsley and spring onions.

399 Kcal/1682 KJ • 24.3 g Protein • 48.8 g Carbohydrate, of which: 1.4 g sugars • 13.2 g Fat, of which: 2.9 g saturates • 0.1 g Sodium • 8.1 g Dietary Fibre

●

PERSIAN RICE

SERVES 4

225 g (8 oz) basmati rice • large handful parsley, chopped

large handful coriander, chopped • handful tarragon, chopped

handful mint, chopped • ground black pepper

Gently cook the rice in a pan of boiling water for 8 minutes, then drain. Return the rice to the pan, add the herbs and black pepper. Cover the pan and leave for 5 minutes without removing the lid. Serve.

202 Kcal/845 KJ • 4.2 g Protein • 44.9 g Carbohydrate, of which: no sugars • 0.3 g Fat, of which: no saturates • no Sodium • no Dietary Fibre

MEXICAN BEANS AND RICE

SERVES 4

10 ml (2 tsp) sunflower oil • 1 large onion, peeled and chopped
1 green chilli, deseeded and chopped • 225 g (8 oz) long grain rice
2 tomatoes, skinned and deseeded
750 ml (1¼ pint) vegetable stock
100 g (3½ oz) pinto or red kidney beans, cooked
ground black pepper

Heat the oil in a non-stick fry pan and cook the onion until soft, about 5 minutes. Add the chilli and rice and cook for a further 2 minutes or until the rice turns opaque. Chop the tomatoes and add to the rice. Pour in the stock, bring to the boil, cover and simmer for 10 minutes. Add the beans and black pepper, adding extra water if necessary. Cook for a further 5 minutes. Drain and serve.

*264 Kcal/1120 KJ • 6.8 g Protein • 57.1 g Carbohydrate, of which: 4.0 g sugars •
2.5 g Fat, of which: 0.4 g saturates • 0.2 g Sodium • 4.3 g Dietary Fibre*

PASTA AND NOODLES

●

WHOLEMEAL PASTA SALAD

SERVES 4

1 lettuce, washed and dried • 450 g (1 lb) cooked wholemeal pasta

225 g (8 oz) sweetcorn • 350 g (12 oz) white crab meat

1 apple, cored and diced • 2 tomatoes, chopped

1 courgette, sliced • large handful basil, chopped (optional)

60 ml (4 tbsp) French Dressing (see page 205)

ground black pepper

Line a salad bowl with the lettuce. Mix together the remaining ingredients and place in the centre of the lettuce lined bowl.

336 Kcal/1409 KJ • 23.9 g Protein • 34.4 g Carbohydrate, of which 12.0 g sugars • 12.4 g Fat, of which: 1.6 g saturates • 0.5 g Sodium • 5.6 g Dietary Fibre

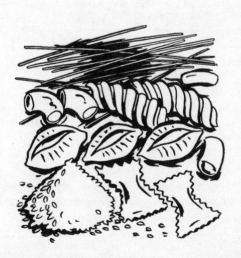

PASTA, BEAN AND VEGETABLE SOUP

SERVES 4

10 ml (2 tsp) olive oil
1 large onion, peeled and chopped
2 carrots, peeled and diced
2 sticks celery, chopped
1 clove garlic, crushed
4 stalks parsley
2 sprigs thyme
1 bay leaf
1 piece lemon rind
225 g (8 oz) white cabbage, finely sliced
100 g (3 1/2 oz) frozen peas
400 g (14 oz) chopped tinned tomatoes
150 g (5 oz) tomato purée
400 g (14 oz) cooked haricot beans
175 g (6 oz) macaroni
2 rashers lean back bacon, cut into small pieces
ground black pepper
750 ml (1 1/4 pint) water

Heat the oil in a large saucepan and cook the onion, carrot and celery until soft, about 8 minutes. Add the garlic and cook for a further 2 minutes. Tie the parsley, thyme, bay leaf and lemon rind together with a piece of string to make a bouquet garni. Add the cabbage, peas, tomatoes, tomato purée, beans, macaroni, bacon, black pepper and bouquet garni to the pan with the water. Bring to the boil and simmer for 20 minutes. Remove the bouquet garni and serve.

411 Kcal/1729 KJ • 20.5 g Protein • 63.6 g Carbohydrate, of which 14.4 g sugars • 10.1 g Fat, of which: 3.0 g saturates • 0.3 g Sodium • 17.3 g Dietary Fibre

●

PASTA WITH KIDNEY BEANS AND BACON

SERVES 4

10 ml (2 tsp) sunflower oil
1 large onion, peeled and chopped
1 clove garlic, crushed
1.25 ml ($1/4$ tsp) chilli powder
225 g (8 oz) wholemeal pasta
400 g (14 oz) can kidney beans, drained
400 g (14 oz) can chopped tomatoes
100 g (4 oz) lean bacon, chopped into bite-sized pieces
200 g (7 oz) can sweetcorn, drained
7.5 ml ($1/2$ tbsp) tomato purée
ground black pepper
30 ml (2 tbsp) chopped fresh parsley

Heat oil in a pan and cook the onion for about 8 minutes until soft. Add the garlic and chilli powder and fry for 1 minute. Meanwhile cook the pasta in a large pan of boiling water for 10 minutes or until al dente. Drain. When the onion is softened add the beans, tomatoes, bacon, sweetcorn, tomato purée and black pepper. Simmer for 15 minutes. Mix the pasta with the bean sauce and simmer for 5 minutes. Sprinkle with parsley and serve.

---

413 Kcal/1740 KJ • 21.5 g Protein • 72.6 g Carbohydrate, of which 11.4 g sugars • 6.1 g Fat, of which: 1.3 g saturates • 0.7 g Sodium • 14.7 g Dietary Fibre

PASTA AL FUNGHI

SERVES 2

150 g (5 oz) shitake mushrooms
150 g (5 oz) oyster mushrooms
100 g (3 1/2 oz) button mushrooms
15 ml (1 tbsp) olive oil
1 small onion, peeled and finely chopped
1 clove garlic, crushed
1/2 green pepper, deseeded and chopped
225 g (8 oz) fresh pasta
30 ml (2 tbsp) chopped fresh coriander
40 g (1 1/2 oz) pumpkin seeds, toasted (optional)
soy sauce, to serve (optional)

Wipe the mushrooms and slice the large ones. Heat the oil in
a pan and cook the onion, garlic and pepper until browned
and softened, about 5-8 minutes. Add the mushrooms and
continue cooking for 5 minutes (the pan will be full at this
stage but they will cook down). Cook the pasta in a large pan
of boiling water for 7 minutes or until tender. Add enough
water to the mushroom mixture to prevent sticking and cook
for a further 5 minutes. Stir in the coriander. Serve the
mushroom sauce with the freshly cooked pasta. Sprinkle the
pumpkin seeds over the sauce, if using, and dress with a small
amount of soy sauce if liked. Variations: Instead of pasta,
serve the sauce with toasted bread, cooked rice or jacket
potato.

*427 Kcal/1799 KJ • 16.9 g Protein • 46.2 g Carbohydrate, of which 9.3 g sugars
• 20.0 g Fat, of which: 4.5 g saturates • trace Sodium • 10.3 g Dietary Fibre*

PASTA WITH GREEN BEANS AND PRAWNS OR MUSHROOMS

SERVES 4

750 g (1½ lb) French beans, trimmed
225 g (8 oz) egg noodles
7.5 ml (1½ tsp) sunflower oil
2.5 ml (½ tsp) sesame oil
350 g (12 oz) peeled prawns
2 cloves garlic, crushed
45 ml (3 tbsp) soy sauce

Cut the French beans in half. Bring a large pan of water to the boil and add the beans. Cook for 5 minutes or until just tender. Drain. Meanwhile, cook the egg noodles in a large pan of boiling water for 10–12 minutes or according to packet instructions. Drain. Heat the oils in a wok and stir-fry the prawns and garlic for 2 minutes. Add the French beans and noodles and stir for 4 minutes. Sprinkle over the soy sauce.

361 Kcal/1518 KJ • 28.8 g Protein • 44.4 g Carbohydrate, of which 2.6 g sugars • 8.8 g Fat, of which: 0.5 g saturates • 1.5 g Sodium • 8.8 g Dietary Fibre

Variation: Pasta with green beans and mushrooms. Use 350g (12 oz) mushrooms instead of prawns. A mixture of cep and chanterelle mushrooms have a rich flavour but field mushrooms also make a tasty dish. Cook for 5 minutes before adding the noodles and French beans.

278 Kcal/1173 KJ • 10.6 g Protein • 44.4 g Carbohydrate, of which: 2.6 g sugars • 7.7 g Fat, of which: 0.4 g saturates • 0.1 g Sodium • 11.0 g Dietary Fibre

PASTA WITH TOMATO AND AUBERGINE SAUCE

SERVES 4

1 large aubergine, diced • 10 ml (2 tsp) olive oil

1 quantity Tomato Sauce (see page 200) • 85 ml (3 fl oz) red wine

4 anchovy fillets, finely chopped • 25 g (1 oz) capers (optional)

225 g (8 oz) pasta

Heat the oil in a large saucepan and cook the aubergine for 5 minutes, stirring constantly. Cover and cook over a low heat for another 5 minutes or until soft. Add tomato sauce, wine, anchovy fillets and capers, if using, and simmer for 15 minutes. Meanwhile, cook the pasta in a large pan of boiling water for 10 minutes or until al dente. Drain and mix the sauce with the pasta.

276 Kcal/1166 KJ • 8.8 g Protein • 48.2 g Carbohydrate, of which 6.5 g sugars • 5.1 g Fat, of which: 0.7 g saturates • 0.1 g Sodium • 6.2 g Dietary Fibre

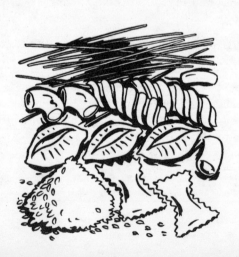

PASTA WITH FRESH TOMATOES

SERVES 4

20 ml (4 tsp) olive oil
10 ml (2 tsp) finely chopped fresh root ginger (optional)
750 g (1½ lb) canned chopped tomatoes or 1 kg (2 lb) extra-ripe tomatoes, skinned and chopped
5 ml (1 tsp) sugar
ground black pepper
225 g (8 oz) pasta

Heat the oil in large saucepan and gently cook the ginger and tomatoes for 10 minutes, stirring frequently. Add the sugar and black pepper. Cook the pasta in a large pan of boiling water for 10 minutes or until al dente. Drain and serve with the sauce.

---

273 Kcal/1158 KJ • 8.5 g Protein • 49.4 g Carbohydrate, of which 7.5 g sugars • 6.0 g Fat, of which: 0.9 g saturates • trace Sodium • 5.6 g Dietary Fibre

PASTA WITH LIVER

SERVES 4

350 g (12 oz) chicken livers, trimmed
10 ml (2 tsp) sunflower oil
1 large onion, peeled and finely chopped
2 cloves garlic, crushed
2 tomatoes, skinned
150 ml ($^1/_4$ pint) chicken stock
sprig sage
ground black pepper
450 g (1 lb) fresh pasta

Cut the chicken livers into large pieces. Heat the oil in a large non stick fry pan and cook the onion and garlic until soft, about 5 – 8 minutes. Stir in the tomatoes and cook for a further 4 minutes. Add the chicken stock and simmer for about 10 minutes. Stir in the chicken livers, sage and black pepper and cook over a gentle heat for 25 minutes or until cooked. Keep uncovered if it starts to stick and add a little water, but the mixture should be fairly thick. Meanwhile, cook the pasta in a large pan of boiling water for about 7 minutes. Drain. Mix the sauce with pasta.

364 Kcal/1536 KJ • 25.1 g Protein • 48.6 g Carbohydrate, of which 6.0 g sugars • 9.1 g Fat, of which: 2.2 g saturates • 0.3 g Sodium • 4.3 g Dietary Fibre

SPICY CHICKEN OR NUTTY NOODLES

SERVES 4

225 g (8 oz) noodles
5 ml (1 tsp) sunflower oil
1 large onion, peeled and chopped
2.5 cm (1 in) piece fresh root ginger, peeled and finely chopped
2 cloves garlic, crushed
15 ml (1 tbsp) curry powder
1 dried red chilli, crushed (optional)
50 ml (2 fl oz) chicken stock
25 ml (1 fl oz) dry sherry
15 ml (1 tbsp) tomato purée
15 ml (1 tbsp) soy sauce
250 g (8 oz) beansprouts
250 g (8 oz) cooked chicken, cut into small pieces

Cook the noodles in a pan of boiling water for 3 minutes. Drain and rinse with cold water. Heat the oil in a wok, and stir-fry the onion and ginger for 4 minutes. Add the garlic, curry powder and chilli, if using, and fry for a further minute. Add the stock, sherry, tomato purée, soy sauce and beansprouts and cook for 4 minutes, stirring frequently. Stir in the chicken and noodles and cook for 4 minutes. Serve.

412 Kcal/1735 KJ • 25.1 g Protein • 51.1 g Carbohydrate, of which 3.1 g sugars • 12.1 g Fat, of which: 1.6 g saturates • 0.2 g Sodium • 3.5 g Dietary Fibre

Variation: Spicy nutty noodles. Use 75 g (3 oz) chopped peanuts instead of the chicken, adding them with the stock.

422 Kcal/1776 KJ • 15.2 g Protein • 52.7 g Carbohydrate, of which 3.7 g sugars • 16.9 g Fat, of which: 1.9 g saturates • 0.1 g Sodium • 5.0 g Dietary Fibre

BEANS AND LENTILS

CHICKEN WITH CHICK PEAS AND APRICOTS

SERVES 4

4 large chicken breasts, each cut into 3 pieces
1 dried red chilli • 1 small cinnamon stick
5 ml (1 tsp) cumin seeds • 4 green cardamom pods • 8 cloves
2.5 cm (1 in) piece fresh root ginger, peeled and finely chopped
2 cloves garlic, crushed • 100 g (4 oz) dried no-soak apricots
150 ml ($^1/_4$ pint) water • 10 ml (2 tsp) sunflower oil
1 large onion, peeled and chopped • 15 ml (1 tbsp) tomato purée
15 ml (1 tbsp) white malt vinegar • 10 ml (2 tsp) sugar
400 g (14 oz) canned chick peas, drained

Place the chicken into a large non-porous bowl. Put the chilli, cinnamon, cumin, cardamom pods and cloves into a spice grinder and grind as fine as possible. Rub half the spice mixture into the chicken with half the ginger and garlic. Set aside for at least 1 hour. Cook the apricots in the water until tender. Leave to cool in the pan. Heat a wok, add the oil and cook the onion for 7 minutes, stirring frequently. Stir in the rest of the ginger and garlic and cook for a further minute. Remove the onion mixture. Add the chicken and cook for 3 minutes until lightly cooked. Add the remaining spice mixture and onion mixture and cook for further 2 minutes. Stir in the tomato purée, vinegar, sugar, chick peas and apricots with the cooking juice. Cook for 15 minutes and serve.

Variations: Use 450 g (1 lb) leg of lamb chops instead of chicken. Cook for 30 minutes instead of 15 minutes at the end of cooking. (Alternatively for the spices, mix together a pinch of chilli powder, 2.5 ml ($^1/_2$ tsp) ground cinnamon, 5ml (1 tsp) ground cumin and 2.5 ml ($^1/_2$ tsp) garam marsala.

> *321 Kcal/1339 KJ • 29.9 g Protein • 36.2 g Carbohydrate, of which: 19.3 g sugars • 7.3 g Fat, of which: 1.8 g saturates • 0.1 g Sodium • 11.9 g Dietary Fibre*

DHAL

SERVES 4

150 g (5 oz) red lentils
1 cm ($^1/_2$ in) piece unpeeled fresh root ginger, thinly sliced
10 ml (2 tsp) sunflower oil
2 large onions, peeled and finely chopped
2.5 ml ($^1/_2$ tsp) ground turmeric • 5 ml (1 tsp) ground cumin
5 ml (1 tsp) ground coriander • 1.25 ml ($^1/_4$ tsp) chilli powder

Place the lentils and ginger in a large saucepan and cover with boiling water. Gently simmer for 30–45 minutes until the lentils are soft. Drain and remove the pieces of ginger. Heat the oil in a non-stick fry pan and gently cook the onions until soft, about 5–8 minutes. Add the spices and cook for a further 2 minutes. Mix the lentils and spices together in a large saucepan and cook over a low heat for 10 minutes, stirring frequently to prevent sticking. Add more water if necessary to prevent sticking. (Dhal should be the consistency of runny porridge).

> *162 Kcal/675 KJ • 9.9 g Protein • 24.8 g Carbohydrate, of which: 4.8 g sugars • 3.2 g Fat, of which: 0.3 g saturates • trace Sodium • 5.4 g Dietary Fibre*

●

K E E M A

SERVES 4

350 g (12 oz) lean minced beef • 5 ml (1 tsp) sunflower oil

1 large onion, peeled and sliced • 1 clove garlic, crushed

5 ml (1 tsp) ground cumin • 5 ml (1 tsp) ground turmeric

1.25 ml (¼ tsp) chilli powder • 225 g (8 oz) frozen peas

15 ml (1 tbsp) tomato purée

Brown the minced beef in a a large non-stick pan, then remove to a large bowl. Heat the oil in the pan and cook the onion until soft, about 8 minutes. Add the garlic and spices and cook for a further 2 minutes. Return the meat to the pan, add the peas, tomato purée and a little water. Cover and simmer for 25 minutes.

175 Kcal/731 KJ • 22.0 g Protein • 7.7 g Carbohydrate, of which: 4.2 g sugars • 6.5 g Fat, of which: 2.0 g saturates • trace Sodium • 7.6 g Dietary Fibre

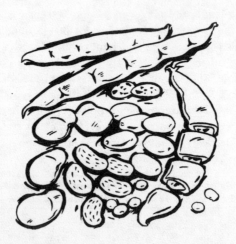

BUTTERBEAN AND MUSHROOM BAKE

SERVES 4

225 g (8 oz) dried butter beans, cooked, or
600 g (1 lb 5 oz) canned butter beans

15 ml (1 tbsp) lemon juice • ground black pepper

5 ml (1 tsp) sunflower oil • 250 g (8 oz) mushrooms, sliced

25 g (1 oz) sunflower margarine • 25 g (1 oz) wholemeal flour

300 ml (½ pint) water • 25 g (1 oz) Cheddar cheese, grated

25 g (1 oz) fresh breadcrumbs

Soak the dried butter beans for at least 4 hours. Drain and cook in a pan of unsalted boiling water for 40–50 minutes or until tender. Drain. If using canned beans, just drain. Put the beans into a large greased ovenproof dish. Add the lemon juice and black pepper. Heat the oil in a pan and fry the mushrooms then add to the dish. Heat the margarine in a non-stick saucepan and add the flour. Cook for 2 minutes over a low heat, stirring, then slowly add the water to make a pouring sauce. Pour over the butter beans and mushrooms. Sprinkle with cheese and breadcrumbs. Cook, in the oven at 180°C (350°F) mark 4 for 25 minutes.

275 Kcal/1147 KJ • 14.9 g Protein • 34.6 g Carbohydrate, of which: 2.6 g sugars • 9.6 g Fat, of which: 2.8 g saturates • 0.2 g Sodium • 10.1 g Dietary Fibre

●

LAZY LENTILS

SERVES 4

175 g (6 oz) red lentils • 100 g (3$\frac{1}{2}$ oz) Cheddar cheese, grated

5 ml (1 tsp) vegetable extract • 5 ml (1 tsp) dried mixed herbs

10 ml (2 tsp) sunflower oil • 2 medium onions, peeled and chopped

1 clove garlic, crushed • 300 ml ($\frac{1}{2}$ pint) water

Put the lentils, cheese, vegetable extract and mixed herbs into a bowl. Heat the oil in a non-stick pan and gently fry the onions and garlic. Mix with the lentils and spoon into a large lightly greased ovenproof dish. Add the water and cover the dish with foil. Cook in the oven at 180°C (350°F) mark 4 for 1$\frac{1}{2}$ hours.

261 Kcal/1085 KJ • 16.7 g Protein • 24.1 g Carbohydrate, of which: 4.8 g sugars • 11.5 g Fat, of which: 5.8 g saturates • 0.3 g Sodium • 5.4 g Dietary Fibre

●

LENTIL BOBOTIE

SERVES 4

10 ml (2 tsp) sunflower oil • 2 medium onions, peeled and chopped

1 clove garlic, crushed • 15 ml (1 tbsp) curry powder

50 g (2 oz) sultanas • 5 ml (1 tsp) dried mixed herbs

250 g (8 oz) red lentils • 300 ml ($\frac{1}{2}$ pint) skimmed milk

15 ml (1 tbsp) vinegar • ground black pepper • pinch salt

Heat the oil in a pan and gently fry the onions for 8 minutes. Add the garlic and fry for a further 2 minutes. Mix all the ingredients together in a bowl. Place the mixture in a large greased ovenproof dish and cover with foil. Cook in the oven at 180°C (350°F) mark 4 for 1$\frac{3}{4}$ hours.

289 Kcal/1210 KJ • 18.4 g Protein • 49.7 g Carbohydrate, of which: 18.0 g sugars • 3.2 g Fat, of which: 0.4 g saturates • trace Sodium • 9.3 g Dietary Fibre

●

HUMMUS

SERVES 4

250 g (8 oz) chick peas, cooked • 75 ml (5 tbsp) lemon juice

30 ml (2 tbsp) tahini • 1–2 cloves garlic, crushed

salt • pinch ground cumin

Purée the chick peas, lemon juice, tahini and garlic in a food processor until soft. Season and add water, if necessary.

225 Kcal/940 KJ • 13.4 g Protein • 32.1 g Carbohydrate, of which: 2.7 g sugars • 6.0 g Fat, of which: no saturates • trace Sodium • 13.5 g Dietary Fibre

●

BLACK BEAN SOUP

SERVES 4

175 g (6 oz) black beans, soaked • 10 ml (2 tsp) sunflower oil

1 large onion, peeled and chopped • 4 sticks celery, chopped

2 carrots, peeled and chopped • 1 clove garlic, crushed

5 ml (1 tsp) ground cumin • ground black pepper

pinch chilli powder (optional)

1.5 litres (2^{1}/$_{2}$ pints) vegetable stock

Soak the beans overnight in water. Alternatively place the beans in a large pan, cover with water and bring to the boil cook for 2 minutes, then turn off the heat and leave for 1 hour. Heat in oil in a large saucepan and sauté the onion, celery and carrots for 8 minutes. Add the garlic and spices and cook for a further 2 minutes. Drain the beans, add to the pan with the stock and simmer for 2 hours or until the beans are cooked. Alternatively, the soup can be cooked in a pressure cooker for 45 minutes. Purée the soup in a blender.

179 Kcal/748 KJ • 10.3 g Protein • 27.1 g Carbohydrate, of which: 5.3 g sugars • 3.2 g Fat, of which: 0.3 g saturates • 0.2 g Sodium • 4.1 g Dietary Fibre

PORK AND BEAN
OR COURGETTE
AND BEAN GOULASH

SERVES 4

350 g (12 oz) pork fillet, trimmed of fat • 15 ml (1 tbsp) soya oil
2 large onions, peeled and chopped
1 green pepper, deseeded and chopped
1 clove garlic, crushed • 15 ml (1 tbsp) paprika • sprig of thyme
400 g (14 oz) can chopped tomatoes • 15 ml (1 tbsp) tomato purée
400 g (14 oz) cooked kidney beans • 75 ml (5 tbsp) water

Cut the pork into medium-sized pieces. Heat the oil and brown the meat. Remove from the pan. Gently fry the onions and pepper in the pan for 5 minutes or until soft. Add the garlic and cook for a further minute. Stir in the paprika and thyme and cook for 2 minutes. Return the meat to the pan with the tomatoes, tomato purée, kidney beans and water. Gently simmer for 1 hour.

286 Kcal/1197 KJ • 27.7 g Protein • 25.2 g Carbohydrate, of which: 7.9 g sugars • 9.1 g Fat, of which: 2.7 g saturates • 0.1 g Sodium • 9.6 g Dietary Fibre

Variation: Courgette and bean goulash. For a vegetarian version, use 450 g (1 lb) courgettes instead of the meat, adding them with the garlic.

186 Kcal/777 KJ • 11.4 g Protein • 30.2 g Carbohydrate, of which: 7.8 g sugars • 3.4 g Fat, of which: 0.3 g saturates • trace Sodium • 9.6 g Dietary Fibre

VEGETABLE CHILLI

SERVES 4

15 ml (1 tbsp) olive oil
2 medium onions, peeled and chopped
2 cloves garlic, crushed
225 g (8 oz) carrots, peeled and chopped into chunky sticks
1 large red pepper, deseeded and sliced
100 g (3$^{1}/_{2}$ oz) mushrooms, chopped into chunky pieces
5 ml (1 tsp) ground cumin
5 ml (1 tsp) dried oregano
2.5 ml ($^{1}/_{2}$ tsp) cayenne pepper
10 ml (2 tsp) mild chilli seasoning
225 g (8 oz) can tomatoes
75 g (3 oz) tomato purée
225 g (8 oz) cooked kidney beans
225 g (8 oz) cooked haricot beans
1 bay leaf   300 ml ($^{1}/_{2}$ pint) vegetable stock
ground black pepper

Heat the oil in a large pan and cook the onions until soft, about 5–8 minutes. Add the garlic and fry for a further minute. Stir in the vegetables, cover the pan and cook for 2 minutes. Add all the remaining ingredients and simmer for 20 minutes. Remove the bay leaf and serve.

216 Kcal/905 KJ • 12.1 g Protein • 31.2 g Carbohydrate, of which: 11.5 g sugars • 5.7 g Fat, of which: 0.7 g saturates • 0.3 g Sodium • 13.2 g Dietary Fibre

BEAN PÂTÉ

SERVES 4

15 ml (1 tbsp) sunflower oil
1 onion, peeled and chopped
1 clove garlic, crushed
1.25 ml (¼ tsp) ground cumin
1.25 – 2.5 ml (¼ – ½ tsp) Tabasco sauce
400 g (14 oz) can red kidney beans, drained
100 ml (4 fl oz) water
30 ml (2 tbsp) Greek yogurt
paprika

Heat the oil in a pan and gently cook the onion until well browned, about 10–12 minutes. Add the garlic, cumin and Tabasco sauce. Stir in the beans and water, then cook down to a thickened mixture, mashing the beans slightly so that it is fairly smooth. Transfer the pâté to a serving bowl. Spread the yogurt over the top and lightly sprinkle with paprika.

392 Kcal/1638 KJ • 24.0 g Protein • 61.2 g Carbohydrate, of which: 3.7 g sugars • 5.1 g Fat, of which: 0.8 g saturates • trace Sodium • 5.0 g Dietary Fibre

LENTIL AND SPINACH SOUP

SERVES 4

175 g (6 oz) green lentils
10 ml (2 tsp) soya oil
1 large onion, peeled and chopped
5 ml (1 tsp) ground cumin
450 g (1 lb) fresh, thawed or frozen spinach, washed
300 ml (¹/₂ pint) vegetable stock
ground black pepper

Cover the lentils with water in a large saucepan. Bring to the boil and simmer for 40 minutes. Heat the oil in a non-stick fry pan and cook the onion until just soft, about 5 minutes. Add the cumin and cook for a further 2 minutes. Stir in the spinach and cook until it becomes limp. Drain the lentils and mix with the spinach and stock. Purée the soup in a blender. Reheat, add black pepper to taste and serve.

206 Kcal/862 KJ • 15.4 g Protein • 31.0 g Carbohydrate, of which: 4.0 g sugars • 3.6 g Fat, of which: 0.4 g saturates • 0.3 g Sodium • 5.9 g Dietary Fibre

BEAN SALAD (PLUS TUNA OR BACON)

SERVES 4

350 g (12 oz) French beans, trimmed
400 g (14 oz) cooked red kidney beans
225 g (8 oz) cooked chick peas • Dressing:
15 ml (1 tbsp) Greek yogurt
large pinch sugar
ground black pepper
15 ml (1 tbsp) chopped fresh mint (optional)
5 ml (1 tsp) French mustard
15 ml (1 tbls) olive oil
15 ml (1 tbsp) red wine vinegar

Steam the French beans until just tender, about 7 minutes. Put all the beans and chick peas into a large salad bowl. Mix together the dressing ingredients and pour over the beans. Toss to mix together. Allow to stand for 1 hour to let the flavours mix before serving.

• 57 Kcal/657 KJ • 9.9 g Protein • 21.8 g Carbohydrate, of which: 3.2 g sugars • 4.1 g Fat, of which: 0.6 g saturates • trace Sodium • 11.3 g Dietary Fibre

Variations: Tuna and Bean Salad: Add 200 g (7 oz) canned tuna, drained and flaked, to the salad.

217 Kcal/909 KJ • 23.4 g Protein • 21.8 g Carbohydrate, of which: 3.2 g sugars • 4.7 g Fat, of which: 0.6 g saturates • trace Sodium • 11.3 g Dietary Fibre

Bacon and Bean Salad: 100 g (4 oz) lean back bacon. Grill. Cut into small pieces and add to the salad.

230 Kcal/962 KJ • 17.5 g Protein • 21.8 g Carbohydrate, of which: 3.2 g sugars • 8.8 g Fat, of which: 2.5 g saturates

VEGETABLES

MUSHROOMS À LA GRECQUE

SERVES 4

10 ml (2 tsp) olive oil
1 small onion, peeled and finely chopped
1 clove garlic, crushed
150 g (5 oz) tomato purée
300 ml ($^1/_2$ pint) water
1 bay leaf
60 ml (4 tbsp) chopped fresh parsley
10 coriander seeds, tied inside a muslin bag or coffee filter bag to make a bouquet garni
ground black pepper
750 g (1$^1/_2$ lb) mushrooms, thickly sliced

Heat the oil in a pan and gently fry the onion until soft, about 5 minutes. Add the garlic and cook for a further minute. Add the remaining ingredients, except the mushrooms, and simmer for 30 minutes. Add the mushrooms and a little water if necessary, then cook for a further 15 minutes. Remove the bouquet garni before serving.

76 Kcal/316 KJ • 4.6 g Protein • 5.4 g Carbohydrate, of which: 5.0 g sugars •
4.1 g Fat, of which: 0.6 g saturates • trace Sodium • 3.0 g Dietary Fibre

STIR-FRY VEGETABLES
(WITH CHICKEN OR PORK)

SERVES 4

10 ml (2 tsp) sunflower oil
1 large onion, peeled and chopped
2 carrots, peeled and cut into fine matchsticks
2.5 cm (1 inch) piece fresh root ginger, peeled and finely chopped
1 clove garlic, crushed
275 g (10 oz) chicken breast or pork fillet, cut into fine strips (optional)
1/4 white cabbage, finely chopped
100 g (3 1/2 oz) mushrooms, sliced
250 g (8 oz) beansprouts
15 ml (1 tbsp) dry sherry
30 ml (2 tbsp) soy sauce

Heat the oil in a wok or large non-stick fry pan and stir-fry the onion, carrots and ginger for 3 minutes, stirring continuously. Add the garlic and stir for another minute. If using chicken or pork, remove the vegetables from the pan and fry the meat for 3 minutes. Return the vegetables to the pan with the cabbage, mushrooms and beansprouts, and stir-fry for 2 minutes. Add the sherry and soy sauce, then cover and cook for 4 minutes.

VEGETABLES ONLY
71 Kcal/297 KJ • 4.1 g Protein • 7.4 g Carbohydrate, of which: 2.3 g sugars •
2.8 g Fat, of which: 0.4 g saturates • trace Sodium • 2.3 g Dietary Fibre

---

WITH CHICKEN OR PORK
155 Kcal/645 KJ • 18.2 g Protein • 7.4 g Carbohydrate, of which: 2.3 g sugars •
5.8 g Fat, of which: 1.3 g saturates • trace Sodium • 2.3 g Dietary Fibre

---

MANGE TOUT AND CARROTS WITH SOY SAUCE

SERVES 4

300 g (10 oz) baby carrots
350 g (12 oz) mange tout trimmed
30 ml (2 tbsp) soy sauce
1/2 clove garlic, crushed (optional)
1 cm (1/2 in) piece fresh root ginger, peeled and chopped (optional)
25 g (1 oz) sunflower seeds, toasted

Remove the tops from the carrots, then scrub them. Bring a large steamer to the boil and steam the carrots for 5 minutes. Add the mange tout and steam for a further 2 minutes. Place the vegetables, soy sauce, garlic and ginger in a large pan and stir for 1 minute until thoroughly mixed. Put into a large bowl and sprinkle with the sunflower seeds.

97 Kcal/404 KJ • 7.3 g Protein • 10.0 g Carbohydrate, of which: 4.7 g sugars • 3.4 g Fat, of which: 0.1 g saturates • 0.2 g Sodium • 14.1 g Dietary Fibre

S T U F F E D   P E P P E R S

SERVES 4

4 large green peppers, cut in half and deseeded
10 ml (2 tsp) olive oil
2 onions, peeled and chopped
2 cloves garlic, crushed
45 ml (3 tbsp) tomato purée
60 ml (4 tbsp) red wine
75 g (3 oz) cashew nuts
400 g (14 oz) can tomatoes
15 ml (2 tbsp) chopped fresh parsley
15 ml (1 tbsp) chopped fresh thyme
ground black pepper
225 g (8 oz) cooked long grain brown rice

Bring a large pan of water to the boil, then parboil the peppers for 5 minutes. Drain and cool quickly. Put into a large greased ovenproof dish. Heat the oil in a large non-stick pan and fry the onions for 8 minutes or until soft. Add the garlic and cook for a further 2 minutes. Add the remaining ingredients, except the rice, and simmer for 20 minutes. Add the rice and thoroughly mix. Stuff the peppers with the mixture. Place any extra mixture around the peppers. Cook in the oven at 180°C (350°F) mark 4 for 25 minutes.

---

288 Kcal/1212 KJ • 8.9 g Protein • 36.2 g Carbohydrate, of which: 10.8 g sugars • 12.5 g Fat, of which: 0.4 g saturates • trace Sodium • 4.2 g Dietary Fibre

VEGETABLE CURRY

SERVES 4

15 ml (3 tsp) sunflower oil
1 large onion, peeled and chopped
2 celery sticks, chopped
2 cloves garlic, crushed
4 cloves
4 whole green cardamoms
5 ml (1 tsp) ground cumin
2.5 ml ($^1/_2$ tsp) ground coriander
2.5 ml ($^1/_2$ tsp) ground turmeric
5 ml (1 tsp) paprika
pinch chilli powder
5 ml (1 tsp) garam marsala
1 parsnip, peeled and chopped
450 g (1 lb) potatoes, scrubbed and chopped
1 courgette, sliced
$^1/_2$ small cauliflower, broken into florets
100 g ($3^1/_2$ oz) frozen peas
400 g (14 oz) can chopped tomatoes
ground black pepper
60 ml (4 tbsp) water

Heat 5 ml (1 tsp) oil in a large flameproof casserole and cook the onion and celery over a low heat for 10 minutes. Add the garlic and cloves and cook for a further 2 minutes. Add the remaining oil and spices and cook for 2 minutes. Mix in the vegetables, black pepper and water, and cook gently over a low heat for 35–40 minutes until tender.

205 Kcal/855 KJ • 6.9 g Protein • 36.6 g Carbohydrate, of which: 7.1 g sugars •
4.7 g Fat, of which: 0.5 g saturates • trace Sodium • 7.8 g Dietary Fibre

GRILLED SUMMER VEGETABLES

SERVES 4

2 small aubergines
3 courgettes
1 yellow pepper, deseeded
1 red pepper, deseeded
15 ml (1 tbsp) olive oil
15 ml (1 tbsp) wine vinegar
1 clove garlic, crushed
5 ml (1 tsp) chopped fresh oregano
ground black pepper

Cut the aubergine into 0.5 ($^{1}/_{4}$ inch) slices. Cut the courgettes diagonally into 1 cm ($^{1}/_{2}$ inch) slices. Cut the peppers into large slices. Mix the oil, vinegar, garlic, oregano and black pepper in a large bowl. Add the vegetables, cover with the mixture and leave to marinate for at least 1 hour. Cook the vegetables on a barbecue or under a hot grill until just tender, basting frequently.

95 Kcal/398 KJ • 3.5 g Protein • 11.7 g Carbohydrate, of which: 7.0 g sugars •
4.5 g Fat, of which: 0.6 g saturates • trace sodium • 5.2 g Dietary Fibre

SPINACH AND CHEESE SQUARES

SERVES 4

2 large eggs, size 1 or 2 • 100 g (3¹/₂ oz) wholemeal flour

275 g (10 oz) frozen chopped spinach, thawed and drained well

450 g (1 lb) cottage cheese

175 g (6 oz) reduced-fat Cheddar cheese • ground black pepper

Beat the eggs and wholemeal flour together in a large bowl. Add the spinach, cottage cheese, Cheddar cheese and black pepper. Spoon the mixture into a well-greased large ovenproof dish. Bake in the oven at 180°C (350°F) mark 4 for about 45 minutes. Leave to cool for at least 5 minutes before serving.

329 Kcal/1385 KJ • 36.2 g Protein • 22.2 g Carbohydrate, of which: 4.2 g sugars • 11.5 g Fat, of which: 5.5 g saturates • 0.8 g Sodium • 2.2 g Dietary Fibre

GREEN BEANS WITH ALMONDS

SERVES 4

450 g (1 lb) French green beans, topped and tailed

5 ml (1 tsp) sunflower oil • 25 g (1 oz) flaked almonds

Bring a large pan of water to the boil. Parboil the beans for 3 minutes, then drain and cool. Heat the oil in a wok or large non-stick fry pan and stir the beans for 4 minutes. Add the almonds and stir for a further 3 minutes.

54 Kcal/227 KJ • 2.0 g Protein • 1.5 g Carbohydrate, of which: 1.2 g sugars • 5.0 g Fat, of which: 0.4 g saturates • trace Sodium • 4.5 g Dietary Fibre

VEGETABLE AND FISH KEBABS

SERVES 4

1 red pepper, deseeded and cut into chunks
1 green pepper, deseeded and cut into chunks
3 small courgettes, cut into 2.5 cm (1 inch) chunks
225 g (8 oz) cherry tomatoes • 150 (5 oz) button mushrooms
450 g (1 lb) fish, such as monkfish, red mullet, plaice, scallops, baby squid, large raw prawns and langoustine
30 ml (2 tbsp) olive oil • 30 ml (2 tbsp) lemon juice
30 ml (2 tbsp) chopped fresh basil • ground black pepper

For best results, partially cook the peppers and courgettes first by blanching in boiling water for a couple of minutes. Drain and cool. Cut the fish into bite-sized pieces. Thread all the vegetables and fish on to skewers, alternating them. Mix the oil, lemon juice, basil and black pepper together. Heat the grill or barbecue. When hot, cook the kebabs for about 10 minutes, basting liberally with the oil mixture.

---

207 Kcal/867 KJ • 24.6 g Protein • 7.7 g Carbohydrate, of which: 2.5 g sugars • 7.3 g Fat, of which: 1.0 g saturates • 0.2 g Sodium • 2.1 g Dietary Fibre

PEPPER AND POTATO TORTILLA

SERVES 1

2 eggs
10 ml (2 tsp) water • ground black pepper
10 g (¹/₃ oz) sunflower margarine
75 g (3 oz) cooked potato, sliced
50 g (2 oz) red pepper, chopped

Break the eggs into a bowl, add the water and black pepper and beat lightly. Heat the margarine in a 15 cm (6 in) omelette pan until slightly smoking, Add the eggs and proceed as for an ordinary omelette. Preheat the grill. While the omelette is still slightly moist, cover the top with the potato and red pepper. Place the omelette under the grill and brown.

320 Kcal/1329 KJ • 17.0 g Protein • 15.9 g Carbohydrate, of which: 1.4 g sugars • 21.4 g Fat, of which: 5.7 g saturates • 0.3 g Sodium • 1.2 g Dietary Fibre

ITALIAN CABBAGE

SERVES 4

1 head white cabbage, chopped
2.5 ml (¹/₂ tsp) grated nutmeg

Bring a large saucepan of water to the boil. Add the cabbage and cook for 3 – 4 minutes. Drain and sprinkle with the nutmeg before serving.

45 Kcal/190 KJ • 4.8 g Protein • 6.8 g Carbohydrate, of which: 6.2 g sugars • 0.2 g Fat, of which: no saturates • trace Sodium • 7.9 g Dietary Fibre

POPPY SEED LEEKS

SERVES 4

4 large leeks, washed and sliced • 5 ml (1 tsp) sunflower oil

15 ml (1 tbsp) poppy seeds • ground black pepper

Steam the leeks for 3 minutes. Drain. Heat the oil in a wok and cook the poppy seeds for 30 seconds. Add the leeks and black pepper and cook for a further 2 minutes, stirring constantly.

42 Kcal/175 KJ • 2.2 g Protein • 5.4 g Carbohydrate, of which: 5.2 g sugars • 1.5 g Fat, of which: 0.2 g saturates • trace Sodium • 4.4 g Dietary Fibre

GREEN BEANS IN TOMATO SAUCE

SERVES 4

450 g (1 lb) runner beans • 15 ml (1 tbsp) olive oil

1 medium onion, peeled and chopped • 2 cloves garlic, crushed

200 g (7 oz) canned tomatoes • 150 ml (1 tbsp) tomato purée

100 ml (4 fl oz) water • large handful parsley, chopped

large pinch sugar • ground black pepper

Top and tail the beans and remove any strings, if necessary. Cut into 5 cm (2 in) pieces. Heat the oil in a pan and gently cook the onion until soft, about 5 minutes. Add the garlic and cook for a further 2 minutes. Stir in the tomatoes, tomato purée, water, parsley, sugar and black pepper then cover and simmer for 25 minutes. Add the green beans and cook for a further 15–20 minutes until the beans are tender. Serve hot or cold as a starter.

64 Kcal/268 KJ • 2.0 g Protein • 6.1 g Carbohydrate, of which: 5.4 g sugars • 3.8 g Fat, of which: 0.5 g saturates • trace Sodium • 4.8 g Dietary Fibre

AUBERGINE PÂTÉ

SERVES 4

2 medium aubergines

2 cloves garlic, crushed

15 ml (1 tbsp) oil

30 ml (2 tbsp) pomegranate juice or orange juice

2.5 ml (½ tsp) paprika

pinch chilli seasoning

Prick the aubergines with a fork and place on a baking tray.
Bake in the oven at 180°C (350°F) mark 4 for 30 minutes or
until tender. When the aubergines are cooked, remove the
skin while hot. Purée the flesh in a food processor with the
garlic, oil, pomegranate juice, paprika and chilli. Leave to
cool, then serve with pitta bread.

*66 Kcal/278 KJ • 1.4 g Protein • 7.1 g Carbohydrate, of which: 6.0 g sugars •
3.9 g Fat, of which: 0.5 g saturates• trace Sodium • 4.4 g Dietary Fibre*

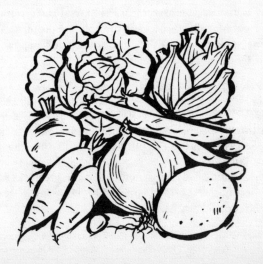

●

SPINACH AND LENTIL OR CHICKEN DHANSAK

SERVES 4

10 ml (2 tsp) sunflower oil • 1 large onion, peeled and chopped
2 cloves garlic, crushed
1 green chilli, deseeded and finely chopped
7.5 ml (1½ tsp) ground cumin • 5 ml (1 tsp) ground coriander
5 ml (1 tsp) garam marsala • 4 cardamoms, crushed
5 ml (1 tsp) ground turmeric • pinch chilli powder
100 g (3½ oz) red lentils • 5 tomatoes, skinned and chopped
300 ml (½ pint) water
450 g (1 lb) fresh spinach, washed, or frozen spinach
large handful coriander, chopped • small handful mint, chopped
ground black pepper

Heat the oil in a large flameproof casserole and gently cook the onion for 10 minutes or until brown. Add the garlic, chilli and spices, and cook for a further 2 minutes. Stir in the lentils, tomatoes and water, and simmer for 30 minutes, stirring occasionally to prevent the mixture from sticking. Add the spinach, coriander, mint and black pepper and simmer for a further 10 minutes.

167 Kcal/699 KJ • 11.4 g Protein • 24.7 g Carbohydrate, of which: 5.5 g sugars • 3.7 g Fat, of which: 0.3 g saturates • 0.1 g Sodium • 4.8 g Dietary Fibre

Variation: Chicken Dhansak. Add 1 small chicken breast per person. Brown the chicken breasts and add at the same time as the lentils.

283 Kcal/1184 KJ • 33.2 g Protein • 24.7 g Carbohydrate, of which: 5.5 g sugars • 6.9 g Fat, of which: 1.4 g saturates • 0.2 g Sodium • 4.8 g Dietary Fibre

TOMATO AND COURGETTE SOUP

SERVES 4

---

10 ml (2 tsp) sunflower oil • 1 large onion, peeled and chopped

2 cloves garlic, crushed • 400 g (14 oz) can tomatoes

450 g (1 lb) courgettes • 450 ml ($^3/_4$ pint) water

30 ml (2 tbsp) tomato purée • 5 ml (1 tsp) sugar

large handful basil, chopped • 15 ml (1 tbsp) wine vinegar

ground black pepper

Heat the oil in a large saucepan and cook the onion and garlic until soft, stirring frequently, about 5–8 minutes. Add the tomatoes, courgettes, water, tomato purée, sugar, basil, vinegar and black pepper. Simmer for 20–25 minutes until all the vegetables are tender. Purée the soup in a blender and serve.

88 Kcal/366 KJ • 4.1 g Protein • 12.5 g Carbohydrate, of which: 7.0 g sugars • 3.0 g Fat, of which: 0.3 g saturates • trace Sodium • 1.8 g Dietary Fibre

CHICKEN WITH WATERCRESS SAUCE

SERVES 4

10 ml (2 tsp) sunflower oil • 4 small chicken breasts
2 medium onions, peeled and chopped • 100 g (3¹/₂ oz) watercress
75 g (3 oz) frozen peas • 175 g (6 oz) peeled old potatoes
450 ml (³/₄ pint) vegetable or chicken stock • ground black pepper

Heat the oil in a large non-stick pan and brown the chicken. Remove the chicken. Add the onions and cook for 5 minutes until just soft. Add the watercress and cook for a further 2 minutes. Return the chicken to the pan and add all the remaining ingredients. Cover and cook for 30 minutes. Remove the chicken and keep warm. Purée the sauce in a blender, then pour over the chicken.

213 Kcal/891 KJ • 24.6 g Protein • 13.8 g Carbohydrate, of which: 4.3 g sugars • 6.9 g Fat, of which: 1.8 g saturates • 0.3 g Sodium • 3.7 g Dietary Fibre

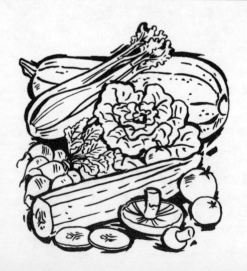

SALAD CRUNCH

●
ITALIAN SALAD

SERVES 4

6 sticks celery, with green leaves removed
100 g (3½ oz) mushrooms, sliced
1 red pepper, deseeded and chopped
large handful parsley, chopped
juice of 1 lemon

Chop the celery and mix together with the other ingredients in a salad bowl.

14 Kcal/60 KJ • 1.3 g Protein • 1.7 g Carbohydrate, of which: 1.7 g sugars • 0.3 g Fat, of which: 0.1 g saturates• trace Sodium • 2.3 g Dietary Fibre

●
FENNEL, APRICOT AND WALNUT SALAD

SERVES 4

1 bulb fennel, with green leaves removed
50 g (2 oz) dried no-soak apricots
25 g (1 oz) walnuts

Chop the fennel, apricots and walnuts. Mix together in a salad bowl.

60 Kcal/250 KJ • 1.8 g Protein • 6.5 g Carbohydrate, of which: 6.3 g sugars • 3.2 g Fat, of which: 0.4 g saturates • trace Sodium • 4.4 g Dietary Fibre

●

MUSHROOM SALAD

SERVES 4

350 g (12 oz) mushrooms, sliced
2 large handfuls chives, chopped
100 g (3½ oz) low-fat natural yogurt
10 ml (2 tsp) lemon juice
ground black pepper

Mix the mushrooms, chives, yogurt, lemon juice and black pepper together in a salad bowl. Leave for 1 hour before serving.

26 Kcal/107 KJ • 2.9 g Protein • 1.9 g Carbohydrate, of which: 1.9 g sugars • 0.7 g Fat, of which: 0.2 g saturates • trace Sodium • 2.2 g Dietary Fibre

●

TURKISH SALAD

SERVES 4

6 tomatoes, cut into small dice
1 cucumber, cut into small dice
1 small mild onion, peeled and finely sliced
large handful mint, chopped
juice of 1 lemon
sprinkling of sumac (optional)

Place the tomatoes, cucumber, onion and mint in a salad bowl. Squeeze the lemon juice over them and mix with the salad. Sprinkle with the sumac to give colour.

22 Kcal/94 KJ • 1.3 g Protein • 4.3 g Carbohydrate, of which: 4.3 g sugars • 0.1 g Fat, of which: trace saturates • trace Sodium • 1.6 g Dietary Fibre

●

WATERCRESS AND ORANGE SALAD

SERVES 4

100 g (3¹/₂ oz) watercress, washed

2 large oranges

Break up the watercress and place in a large salad bowl. Cut off both ends of each orange with a sharp knife. With a small knife, carefully cut off the skin and pith. Cut into thin slices with a bread knife and cut each slice into quarters. Mix the orange pieces with the watercress and serve.

26 Kcal/110 KJ • 1.2 g Protein • 5.7 g Carbohydrate, of which: 5.6 g sugars • no Fat, of which: no saturates • trace Sodium • 2.1 g Dietary Fibre

●

WINTER SALAD

SERVES 4

¹/₂ red cabbage, finely sliced

1 small onion, peeled and finely sliced

1 green pepper, deseeded and finely sliced

1 red pepper, deseeded and finely sliced

45 ml (3 tbsp) French Dressing (see page 205)

Mix all the ingredients together in a large bowl.

107 Kcal/444 KJ • 2.4 g Protein • 5.7 g Carbohydrate, of which: 5.7 g sugars • 8.5 g Fat, of which: 1.2 g saturates • 0.1 Sodium • 4.2 g Dietary Fibre

CARROT AND NUT SALAD

SERVES 4

450 g (1 lb) carrots, peeled

75 g (3 oz) natural roasted peanuts, unsalted

2 large handfuls parsley, chopped

30 ml (2 tbsp) freshly squeezed orange juice

30 ml (2 tbsp) French Dressing (see page 205)

ground black pepper

10 ml (2 tsp) orange flower water (optional)

Grate the carrots. Finely chop the nuts. Mix the nuts with the carrots, parsley, orange juice, dressing, black pepper and orange flower water in a large salad bowl.

185 Kcal/770 KJ • 5.4 g Protein • 8.4 g Carbohydrate, of which: 7.4 g sugars • 14.7 g Fat, of which: 2.5 g saturates • 0.2 Sodium • 4.8 g Dietary Fibre

GARDEN SALAD

SERVES 4

2 handfuls Quattro Stagioni

2 large handfuls red oak leaf lettuce

2 large handfuls Cos lettuce

handful Greek cress

handful rocket

handful coriander leaves

handful parsley leaves

Clean and wash all the salad. Remove and discard any bruised or yellowed leaves, then dry thoroughly. Place in a salad large bowl and serve.

8 Kcal/31 KJ • 0.6 g Protein • 0.8 g Carbohydrate, of which: 0.8 g sugars • 0.3 g Fat, of which: no saturates • trace Sodium • 0.9 g Dietary Fibre

LEMON COLESLAW

SERVES 4

¹/₂ white cabbage
75 g (3 oz) sultanas or raisins
juice of 1 lemon

Finely chop the cabbage and place in a large salad bowl with the sultanas. Squeeze over the lemon juice and mix with the cabbage and sultanas.

65 Kcal/275 KJ • 1.9 g Protein • 15.3 g Carbohydrate, of which: 15.3 g sugars • no Fat, of which: no saturates • trace Sodium • 3.3 g Dietary Fibre

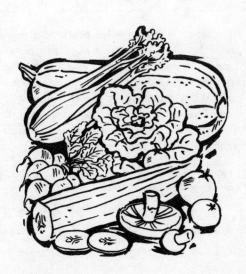

INSALATA DI MARE – SEAFOOD SALAD

SERVES 4

225 g (8 oz) fresh or frozen squid, prepared and cut into rings
100 g (3¹/₂ oz) peeled prawns
225 g (8 oz) unpeeled prawns
large handful parsley, chopped
few leaves basil, chopped
juice of 1 lemon
15 ml (1 tbsp) olive oil
ground black pepper
1 green lettuce
1 red lollo rosso lettuce
2 red peppers, deseeded and sliced
4 tomatoes, sliced

Place the seafood in a large salad bowl. Mix together the parsley, basil, lemon juice, oil and black pepper. Pour over the fish, stir and leave for at least 1 hour in the fridge for the flavours to mix. Remove and discard any bruised or yellowed leaves from the lettuces. Wash and thoroughly dry them. Once the fish has marinated, tear the lettuce into shreds and add to the bowl with the red peppers and tomatoes. Toss, bringing the unpeeled prawns to the surface.

143 Kcal/600 KJ • 19.6 g Protein • 4.2 g Carbohydrate, of which: 4.2 g sugars • 5.4 g Fat, of which: 0.6 g saturates • 0.8 g Sodium • 2.3 g Dietary Fibre

SPINACH AND HAM OR EGG SALAD

SERVES 4

450 g (1 lb) spinach

150 g (5 oz) lean thick-cut honey roast ham

45 ml (3 tbsp) French Dressing (see page 205)

Remove and discard the tough spinach stalks and any bruised or yellowed leaves. Tear the large leaves in half or into thirds. Wash the spinach in at least two changes of water and spin dry. Place the spinach in a large salad bowl. Cut the ham into small bite-sized pieces. Gently heat the French Dressing until just warm, pour over the spinach and toss quickly. Mix in the ham.

148 Kcal/615 KJ • 10.5 g Protein • 4.2 g Carbohydrate, of which: trace sugars • 10.5 g Fat, of which: • 1.8 g saturates • 0.7 Sodium • trace Dietary Fibre

Variation: Instead of the ham add 2 hard-boiled eggs, finely diced.

148 Kcal/614 KJ • 7.4 g Protein • 4.2 g Carbohydrate, of which: trace sugars • 11.9 g Fat, of which: 2.1 g saturates • 0.2 g Sodium • trace Dietary Fibre

THAI CHICKEN SALAD

SERVES 4

2 lettuce
4 small roasted chicken breasts
4 large tomatoes, cut into eighths
1 yellow pepper, deseeded and sliced
6 spring onions, finely sliced
100 g (3½ oz) beansprouts
Dressing:
15 ml (1 tbsp) tahini
15 ml (1 tbsp) sunflower oil
15 ml (1 tbsp) white vinegar
5 ml (1 tsp) sugar
pinch chilli powder

Remove and discard any lettuce leaves that are bruised or yellowed. Wash and thoroughly dry the lettuce, then place in a large salad bowl. Chop the chicken into bite-sized pieces and mix with the tomatoes, pepper, spring onions and beansprouts. Add to the bowl. Mix together the dressing ingredients. Pour over the salad, toss and serve.

---

*237 Kcal/991 KJ • 29 g Protein • 6.4 g Carbohydrate, of which: 4.9 g sugars •
11.0 g Fat, of which: 2.3 g saturates • trace Sodium • 2.1 g Dietary Fibre*

●

SALAD NIÇOISE

SERVES 4

1 – 2 lettuces, depending on size
4 large ripe tomatoes, sliced
225 g (8 oz) French beans, cooked
45 ml (3 tbsp) French Dressing (see page 205)
200 g (7 oz) canned tuna in brine, drained
50 g (2 oz) canned anchovies in oil, drained
2 eggs, hard boiled and halved
12 black olives

Remove and discard any lettuce leaves that are bruised or
yellowed. Wash and thoroughly dry the lettuce, then place in
a large salad bowl. Add the tomatoes, beans and French
Dressing, then gently mix together. Arrange the remaining
ingredients over the top of the salad.

*294 Kcal/221 KJ • 17.0 g Protein • 3.3 g Carbohydrate, of which: 3.2 g sugars •
23.8 g Fat, of which: 4.2 g saturates • 0.6 g Sodium • 4.1 g Dietary Fibre*

AVOCADO, PRAWN OR WALNUT, APPLE AND CELERY SALAD

SERVES 4

2 lettuce
1 avocado, stoned, peeled and diced
350 g (12 oz) peeled prawns
1 apple, cored and diced
$1/2$ bunch of celery, chopped
30 ml (2 tbsp) French Dressing (see page 205)
ground black pepper
juice of 1 lemon

Remove and discard any lettuce leaves that are bruised or yellowed. Wash and thoroughly dry the lettuce, then place in a large salad bowl. Place all the ingredients in the bowl, squeezing over the lemon juice, and toss.

---
247 Kcal/1030 KJ • 22.3 g Protein • 4.7 g Carbohydrate, of which: 4.7 g sugars • 15.7 g Fat, of which: 1.9 g saturates • 1.5 g Sodium • 2.6 g Dietary Fibre
---

Variation: Instead of the prawns use 50 g (2 oz) chopped walnuts in the salad.

---
232 Kcal/963 KJ • 4.1 g Protein • 5.4 g Carbohydrate, of which: 5.1 g sugars • 21.8 g Fat, of which: 2.6 g saturates • 0.1 Sodium • 3.3 g Dietary Fibre
---

DESSERTS

RASPBERRY SORBET

SERVES 4

450 g (1 lb) fresh raspberries or frozen raspberries, thawed
100 g (3¹/₂ oz) caster sugar
150 ml (¹/₄ pint) water
Juice of 1 lemon
1 egg white (optional)

Purée the raspberries and sieve, if preferred. Put the sugar and water in a saucepan and stir over a gentle heat until the sugar has dissolved. Turn up the heat and boil fast for 5 minutes until a sticky syrup forms. When the syrup has cooled, mix it with the fruit purée and lemon juice. Freeze in an ice cream maker for 20 minutes. Alternatively, place the mixture in a bowl in the freezer until beginning to freeze around the edges. Whisk the egg white and fold into the part frozen mixture. Return the sorbet to the freezer until frozen.

Variations. Use other fruit, such as strawberries, blackcurrants, redcurrants, blackberries, gooseberries or kiwi fruit. Alternatively, use the flesh of 2 large ripe mangos, or 450 g (1 lb) rhubarb or 450 g (1 lb) apricots.

---

128 Kcal/538 KJ • 1.1 g Protein • 33.0 g Carbohydrate, of which: 33.0 g sugars • no Fat, of which: no saturates • trace Sodium • 8.3 g Dietary Fibre

ALMOND BISCUITS

MAKES ABOUT 20

These little biscuits will keep for a couple of weeks in an airtight tin, so there is no need to eat them all at once. Alternatively, freeze them for up to 2 months.

150 g (5 oz) ground almonds
150 g (5 oz) caster sugar
25 g (1 oz) plain flour
generous 30 ml (2 tbsp) egg white

Place all the ingredients in a large bowl. Mix together, then knead the paste. If the mixture still seems dry, add a little more egg white. Roll small balls of paste between floured hands. When smooth, place on a greased baking tray and flatten with the back of a fork. Bake in the oven at 180°C (350°F) mark 4 for 10–15 minutes or until just browned underneath.

129 Kcal/544 KJ • 3.1 g Protein • 23.9 g Carbohydrate, of which: 5.8 g sugars •
3.0 g Fat, of which: 0.2 g saturates • trace Sodium • 1.8 g Dietary Fibre

STRAWBERRY YOGURT ICE CREAM

SERVES 4

225 g (8 oz) strawberries
75 g (3 oz) sugar
450 g (16 oz) low-fat natural yogurt
1 egg white (optional)

Purée the strawberries and sugar, then sieve if preferred. Mix with the yogurt. Freeze in an ice cream maker for 20 minutes. Alternatively, place the mixture in the freezer until just beginning to freeze around the edges. Whisk the egg white and fold into the part frozen mixture. Return the ice cream to the freezer until frozen.

152 Kcal/636 KJ • 6.0 g Protein • 32.0 g Carbohydrate, of which: 32.0 g sugars • 1.0 g Fat, of which: no saturates • trace Sodium • 1.2 g Dietary Fibre

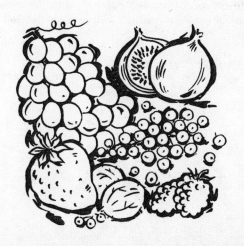

FRESH FRUIT PLATTER

SERVES 4

Selection of fruit such as:

$^1/_2$ watermelon

2 pears

2 peaches

225 g (8 oz) black seedless grapes

plenty of ice cubes

mint leaves for decoration

Cut the melon into small pieces and remove some of the seeds using a small, sharp knife. Cut the pears and peaches in half and remove the stone or core. Cut each piece into three and further divide each piece in half. Crush the ice in a food processor and turn out onto a large serving plate, leaving any water in the processor. Alternatively, put the ice cubes into a thick plastic bag and crush with a rolling pin. Arrange the fruit on top of the ice and decorate with the mint leaves. Serve by giving each person a fork to spear the fruit of their choice.

---

102 Kcal/436 KJ • 1.2 g Protein • 25.9 g Carbohydrate, of which: 25.9 g sugars • no Fat, of which: no saturates • trace Sodium • 2.8 g Dietary Fibre

FRUIT PARCELS

SERVES 4

6 apricots
1 apple, preferably Cox's or Braeburn
$^{1}/_{2}$ small pineapple
200 ml (7 fl oz) apple and mango juice or orange juice

Cut the apricots in half and remove the stone. Cut the apple in half, remove the core, then cut each piece into six. Remove the outside of the pineapple and the core. Cut into thick slices, then cut each slice into three. Arrange a mixture of the fruit onto 23 cm (9 in) squares of foil with grease-proof paper squares on the inside. Divide the fruit juice between the parcels. Fold the foil to completely enclose the fruit. Bake in the oven at 180°C (350°F) mark 4 for 25 minutes. Variation: For a special occasion, substitute 15 ml (1 tbsp) fruit juice with Calvados or brandy.

86 Kcal/359 KJ • 1.2 g Protein • 21.5 g Carbohydrate, of which: 21.5 g sugars • no Fat, of which: no saturates • 3.2 g Sodium • 2.9 g Dietary Fibre

PEACH BRÛLÉE

SERVES 4

6 large fairly ripe peaches
50 ml (2 fl oz) orange juice
125 g (5 oz) Greek yogurt
75 g (3 oz) low-fat natural yogurt
40 – 50 g (1¹/₂ – 2 oz) soft brown sugar, according to size of dish

Remove the skin from the peaches. If the peaches are ripe, simply pull off the skin. Alternatively, skin by cutting a cross in the bottom of each peach and putting into a large bowl of just boiled water. Leave for 4 – 5 minutes, then remove from the bowl and pull off the skin. Cut the peaches in half, then slice and place them in a deep flameproof dish. Pour over the orange juice. Mix together the yogurts. Cover the peaches with the yogurt and sprinkle with the sugar. Heat the grill and place the dish under it. When the sugar has melted and just started to bubble, remove from the grill. Leave to cool. Place in the refrigerator and leave for at least 1 hour.

Variation: For a special occasion, spoon 45 ml (3 tbsp) brandy over the peaches before covering with the yogurt.

142 Kcal/598 KJ • 4.5 g Protein • 26.8 g Carbohydrate, of which: 26.8 g sugars • 2.6 g Fat, of which: 1.5 g saturates • trace Sodium • 1.8 g Dietary Fibre

DRIED FRUIT SALAD

SERVES 4

225 g (8 oz) dried, no-soak fruit
1 cinnamon stick
2 cloves
juice of 1 lemon
1 cooking apple, peeled, cored and sliced
50 g (2 oz) raisins
grated nutmeg

Cover the fruit with water in a pan, then add the cinnamon, cloves and lemon juice. Cook for 10 minutes. Add the apple, raisins and nutmeg and cook for a further 5 minutes. Leave for 10 minutes in the pan before serving.

156 Kcal/658 KJ • 2.4 g Protein • 38.9 g Carbohydrate, of which: 38.8 g sugars • no Fat, of which: no saturates • trace Sodium • 12.5 g Dietary Fibre

PEARS WITH FRESH GINGER

SERVES 4

6 large pears, peeled, cored and sliced
2.5 cm (1 inch) piece fresh root ginger, peeled and grated
150 ml (¼ pint) pineapple juice

Place the pear slices in a bowl. Mix the ginger with the pineapple juice, pour over the pears and serve.

87 Kcal/372 KJ • 0.6 g Protein • 22.5 g Carbohydrate, of which: 22.5 g sugars • no Fat, of which: no saturates • trace Sodium • 3.9 g Dietary Fibre

PEACHES STUFFED WITH ALMONDS

SERVES 4

4 large ripe peaches
50 g (2 oz) ground almonds
25 g (1 oz) caster sugar
1 egg white
100 ml (4 fl oz) orange juice

Remove the stone and skin from the peaches (see page 136 under Peach Brûlée). Place the peaches in a single layer in a deep ovenproof dish. Mix together the almonds, sugar and some of the egg white to form a stiff paste. Using a teaspoon, fill the centre of the peaches with the almond mixture. Pour in the orange juice and cover the dish with foil. Cook in the oven at 190°C (375°F) mark 5 for 25 minutes or until the peaches are tender. Remove cover and cook for a further 5 minutes. Variation: For a special occasion, add 5 ml (1 tsp) of cocoa powder to the almond mixture and use some white wine instead of orange juice.

149 Kcal/628 KJ • 3.7 g Protein • 19.7 g Carbohydrate, of which: 19.7 g sugars • 6.7 g Fat, of which: 0.5 g saturates • trace Sodium • 3.0 g Dietary Fibre

SIMPLE TRIFLE

SERVES 4

350 g (12 oz) fatless sponge
225 g (8 oz) frozen strawberries, thawed
1 large banana
45 ml (3 tbsp) orange juice
250 g (9 oz) Greek yogurt
15 g (½ oz) flaked almonds

Cut the sponge into 5 cm (2 in) squares and place in a medium serving bowl. Place the strawberries on top of the sponge. Peel and slice the banana and place over the strawberries. Pour the orange juice over. Cover the fruit with the yogurt. Sprinkle with flaked almonds and place in the refrigerator for at least 30 minutes before serving.

390 Kcal/1646 KJ • 14.2 g Protein • 57.5 g Carbohydrate, of which: 37.5 g sugars • 13.1 g Fat, of which: 5.2 g saturates • 0.1 g Sodium • 3.4 g Dietary Fibre

BANANA CREAM

SERVES 4

75 g (3 oz) dried no-soak apricots
2 ripe bananas
300 g (10 oz) low-fat yogurt

Chop up the apricots and divide between four ramekins. Purée the bananas with the yogurt in a blender. Divide the yogurt mixture between the ramekins. Serve.

111 Kcal/467 KJ • 5.3 g Protein • 22.3 g Carbohydrate, of which: 21.0 g sugars • 0.8 g Fat, of which: 0.4 g saturates • trace Sodium • 6.0 g Dietary Fibre

WALNUT STUFFED PEARS

SERVES 4

4 large ripe pears, peeled, cored and cut in half
50 g (2 oz) sultanas, roughly chopped
50 g (2 oz) walnuts, finely chopped
40 g (1¹/₂ oz) soft brown sugar
1 egg white
150 ml (¹/₄ pint) pear or apple juice

Place the pears in a greased deep baking dish. Mix together the sultanas, walnuts, brown sugar, egg white and 15 ml (1 tbsp) fruit juice. Spoon the mixture into the pear cavities. Pour over the remainder of the fruit juice and cover the dish with foil. Bake in the oven at 190°C (375°F) mark 5 for 40 minutes or until tender. Remove the foil and cook for a further 5 minutes.

220 Kcal/929 KJ • 3.0 g Protein • 40.2 g Carbohydrate, of which: 40.0 g sugars • 6.4 g Fat, of which: 0.7 g saturates • trace Sodium • 5.4 g Dietary Fibre

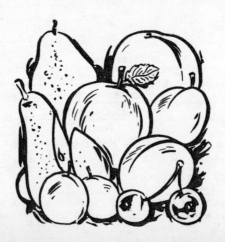

FRUIT KEBABS

SERVES 4

1 banana
1 apple, peeled and cored
$^1/_2$ pineapple
100 g (3$^1/_2$ oz) seedless grapes
10 ml (2 tsp) honey
juice of $^1/_2$ lemon

Peel the banana and cut into four. Cut the apple into bite-sized pieces. Remove the outside of the pineapple, core and cut into bite-sized pieces. Place all the fruit in a large bowl. Mix together the honey and lemon juice. Pour over the fruit and mix together. Thread the fruit on to small bamboo skewers. Serve.

Variations: Use other fruits such as strawberries, apricots, cherries, melon and kiwi fruit. Alternatively serve hot, heat a grill or barbecue and cook the kebabs for 7 minutes. Turn once or twice during the cooking time.

*91 Kcal/382 KJ • 1.0 g Protein • 23.0 g Carbohydrate, of which: 22.3 g sugars •
0.1 g Fat, of which: no saturates • trace Sodium • 2.4 g Dietary Fibre*

CHEESECAKE

SERVES 8

350 g (12 oz) medium-fat curd cheese

100 g (3½ oz) granulated sugar

4 eggs, beaten

25 g (1 oz) plain flour

2.5 ml (½ tsp) baking powder

grated rind and juice of 1 lemon

50 g (2 oz) raisins

Grease a deep 15 cm (6 in) cake tin and line with greaseproof paper. Beat together the cheese and sugar, then gradually add the eggs. Sift the flour and baking powder, and add to the mixture. Stir in the lemon rind, juice and raisins. Pour the mixture into the tin. Bake in the oven at 160°C (325°F) mark 3 for 1 hour or until firm. Serve with a fruit sauce (see page 140).

199 Kcal/832 KJ • 8.3 g Protein • 21.1 g Carbohydrate, of which: 18.7 g sugars • 9.7 g Fat, of which: 4.9 g saturates • trace Sodium • 0.5 g Dietary Fibre

FRUIT SAUCES

Children love dipping pieces of fresh fruit into these sauces. Alternatively, use them instead of cream. For a very special occasion (unless you are trying to lose weight) try the raspberry sauce over chocolate cake! Berry sauces without the yogurt are particularly good served hot.

Nutritional values apply to the whole recipe; not per serving.

MANGO SAUCE

2 mangos
45 ml (3 tbsp) apple or orange juice

Cut the mangos in half and remove the stone with a sharp knife. Peel the mangos, then place the flesh in a blender with the fruit juice. Purée until smooth.

221 Kcal/927 KJ • 2.1 g Protein • 57.0 g Carbohydrate, of which: 57.0 g sugars • no Fat, of which: no saturates • trace Sodium • 4.8 g Dietary Fibre

RASPBERRY SAUCE

150 g (5 oz) raspberries
30 ml (2 tbsp) Greek yogurt

Purée the raspberries and yogurt in a blender. If you want to remove the pips, push the mixture through a sieve.

101 Kcal/420 KJ • 4.9 g Protein • 9.5 g Carbohydrate, of which: 9.5 g sugars • 5.0 g Fat, of which: 2.7 g saturates • trace Sodium • 11.1 g Dietary Fibre

RHUBARB SAUCE

350 g (12 oz) rhubarb
25 g (1 oz) sugar

Cut the ends off the rhubarb and chop into 2.5 cm (1 in)
pieces. Place the rhubarb pieces in a saucepan and just cover
with water. Add the sugar. Bring to the boil and simmer for
about 8 minutes or until mushy. Purée in a blender.
Variation: make with gooseberries, blackberries,
blackcurrants or a mixed fruit sauce of currants and berries.

*120 Kcal/503 KJ • 2.1 g Protein • 29.8 g Carbohydrate, of which: 29.8 g sugars •
no Fat, of which: no saturates • trace Sodium • 9.1 g Dietary Fibre*

BASICS

LEMON MARINADE

Suitable for pork, chicken and fish.

15 ml (1 tbsp) sunflower oil
1 clove garlic, crushed
juice of $^1/_2$ lemon
ground black pepper
30 ml (2 tbsp) chopped fresh herbs or 2.5 ml ($^1/_2$ tsp) dried mixed herbs

Mix all the ingredients together and leave to marinate for at
least 30 minutes. Cook over a barbecue, under a grill or in
the oven at 200°C (400°F) mark 6. **Variation:** Try spices
instead of the herbs.

*142 Kcal/585 KJ • 0.3 g Protein • 1.7 g Carbohydrate, of which: 0.8 g sugars •
15.0 g Fat, of which: 2.0 g saturates • trace Sodium • no Dietary Fibre*

●

YOGURT TANDOORI MARINADE

Suitable for chicken, fish, lamb and beef.

10 ml (2 tsp) sunflower oil
150 ml (5 oz) low-fat natural yogurt
5 ml (1 tsp) ground cumin
1.25 ml ($^1/_4$ tsp) ground turmeric
1.25 ml ($^1/_4$ tsp) chilli powder
5 ml (1 tsp) ground coriander
5 ml (1 tsp) garam marsala
5 ml (1 tsp) paprika
1 large clove garlic, crushed

Mix all the ingredients together and leave to marinate for at least 1 hour. Cook over a barbecue under a grill or in the oven at 230°C (450°F) mark 8.

229 Kcal/953 KJ • 9.7 g Protein • 18.0 g Carbohydrate, of which: 11.3 g sugars • 13.7 g Fat, of which: 2.0 g saturates • 0.1 g Sodium • no Dietary Fibre

SOY SAUCE MARINADE

Suitable for chicken, pork, lamb and beef.

30 ml (2 tbsp) soy sauce
15 ml (1 tbsp) sunflower oil
1 clove garlic, crushed
5 ml (1 tsp) ground cumin
5 ml (1 tsp) ground coriander
ground black pepper

Mix all the ingredients together and leave to marinate for at least 1 hour. Cook over a barbecue, under a grill or in the oven.

Variations: Experiment with other spices.

> *198 Kcal/818 KJ • 3.3 g Protein • 8.1 g Carbohydrate, of which: no sugars*
> *17.2 g Fat, of which: 2.1 g saturates • trace Sodium • no Dietary Fibre*

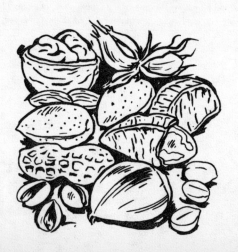

DRIED FRUIT AND NUT STUFFING

5 ml (1 tsp) sunflower oil
1 onion, peeled and chopped
2 small cooking apples, peeled and chopped
5 ml (1 tsp) ground cinnamon
50 g (2 oz) dried no-soak prunes, chopped
50 g (2 oz) dried no-soak apricots, chopped
50 g (2 oz) dried no-soak peaches, chopped
50 g (2 oz) raisins
100 g (4 oz) almonds
45 ml (3 tbsp) water

Heat the oil in a non stick pan and fry the onions until soft, about 5–8 minutes. Add the apples and cook for 3 minutes. Cover and cook for a further 2 minutes. Add the rest of the ingredients and cook for 5 minutes.

1036 Kcal/4351 KJ • 23.0 g Protein • 112.0 g Carbohydrate, of which: 111.0 g sugars • 59.0 g Fat, of which: • 4.9 g saturates • trace Sodium • 43.6 g Dietary Fibre

TOMATO SAUCE

Serve with pasta and hamburgers. Alternatively, add vegetables such as courgettes or aubergines and cook to make a pasta sauce.

10 ml (2 tsp) olive oil
1 medium onion, peeled and chopped
1 clove garlic, crushed
400 g (14 oz) can chopped tomatoes
15 ml (1 tbsp) tomato purée
pinch mixed herbs
pinch sugar
ground black pepper

Heat the oil in a pan and gently brown the onion, over a low heat for about 10 minutes, stirring occasionally. Add the garlic and cook for a further 2 minutes. Stir in the tomatoes, tomato purée, mixed herbs, sugar and black pepper. Cook for 20 minutes or until slightly thickened.

238 Kcal/995 KJ • 7.4 g Protein • 24.3 g Carbohydrate, of which: 24.0 g sugars • 13.0 g Fat, of which: 1.8 g saturates • 0.1 g Sodium • 6.5 g Dietary Fibre

CITRUS SPREAD

1 lemon
100 g (3¹/₂ oz) medium-fat cream cheese
25 g (1 oz) caster sugar

Finely grate the rind from the lemon and mix with the cheese. Squeeze the juice from the lemon. Add 15 ml (1 tbsp) of the lemon juice and the sugar to the cheese. Keep in the refrigerator.

> *561 Kcal/2336 KJ • 18.7 g Protein • 60.1 g Carbohydrate, of which: 60.1 g sugars • 29.0 g Fat, of which: 18.2 g saturates • trace Sodium • no Dietary Fibre*

RAITA

¹/₂ cucumber
150 ml (5 oz) low-fat natural yogurt
pinch paprika

Grate the cucumber and leave to drain in a colander. To speed up the process, use a wooden spoon to press out the moisture. Mix the cucumber with the yogurt and place in a bowl. Sprinkle with paprika.

> *114 Kcal/480 KJ • 9.5 g Protein • 16.7 g Carbohydrate, of which: 16.7 g sugars • 1.5 g Fat, of which: 0.8 g saturates • 0.2 g Sodium • 1.2 g Dietary Fibre*

●

RED PEPPER SAUCE

---

10 ml (2 tsp) sunflower oil • 2 small onions, peeled and chopped

---

2 red peppers, deseeded and chopped

---

couple of sprigs thyme, chopped

---

200 ml (7 fl oz) vegetable stock • ground black pepper

Heat the oil in a pan and gently cook the onions for about 5 minutes until soft. Add the peppers and cook for a further 4 minutes. Stir in the thyme, vegetable stock and black pepper, then cook for 20 minutes. Purée in a blender and serve. Ideal with pasta, grilled pork chops or oven-baked chicken.

---

87 Kcal/360 KJ • 2.0 g Protein • 8.0 g Carbohydrate, of which: 8.0 g sugars • 5.5 g Fat, of which: 0.7 g saturates • trace Sodium • 2.4 g Dietary Fibre

---

●

TOMATO SALSA

---

450 g (1 lb) ripe tomatoes, skinned and deseeded

---

1 small onion, peeled and finely chopped

---

1 – 3 green chillies, deseeded and finely chopped

---

15 ml (1 tbsp) wine vinegar • ground black pepper

---

pinch sugar • 30 ml (2 tbsp) chopped fresh coriander or parsley

---

Finely chop the tomatoes by hand or put in a food processor but be careful not to overblend. Mix with the remaining ingredients. This will keep for up to a week in the refrigerator. **Variation:** Use 400 g (14 oz) can chopped tomatoes in the winter (it doesn't make quite such a good salsa.)

---

182 Kcal/761 KJ • 5.7 g Protein • 18.5 g Carbohydrate, of which: 17.7 g sugars • 10.0 g Fat, of which: 1.4 g saturates • 0.1 g Sodium • 5.2 g Dietary Fibre

---

MANGO AND TOMATO SALSA

1 mango • 225 g (8 oz) ripe tomatoes, skinned and deseeded

1 green chilli, deseeded and finely chopped

15 ml (1 tbsp) chopped fresh mint

15 ml (1 tbsp) chopped fresh coriander

juice of 1 lime • 15 ml (1 tbsp) olive oil

pinch sugar • ground black pepper

Cut the mango in half, take out the stone and remove the skin. Finely chop the mango flesh and tomatoes. Mix with the remaining ingredients.

266 Kcal/1114 KJ • 3.2 g Protein • 35.2 g Carbohydrate, of which: 34.0 g sugars • 13.4 g Fat, of which: 1.8 g saturates • trace Sodium • 5.8 g Dietary Fibre

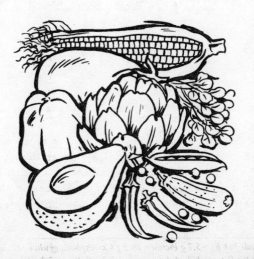

PICA DE GALLO TOMATO RELISH

*Anne first tried this in Jackson, Wyoming. It is a great boost to any
dish but is particularly good with grilled fish, chicken or beef and
warm pitta bread. For those on a diet, it adds flavour without too
many calories!*

$^1/_2$ sweet onion, peeled and finely chopped
2 tomatoes, finely diced
1 – 3 serrano chillies, deseeded and finely chopped
15 ml (1 tbsp) white vinegar
15 ml (1 tbsp) chopped fresh coriander

Combine all the ingredients together in a bowl. Leave for at
least 30 minutes for the flavours to mingle.

*37.7 Kcal/158 KJ • 2.1 g Protein • 7.0 g Carbohydrate, of which: 6.3 g sugars
0.1 g Fat, of which: no saturates • trace Sodium • 2.6 g Dietary Fibre*

FRENCH DRESSING

30 ml (2 tbsp) olive oil
30 ml (2 tbsp) wine or sherry vinegar
2.5 ml (¹/₂ tsp) French mustard
pinch sugar • salt
ground black pepper

Mix all the ingredients together.

Variations: Poppy seed dressing: Add 10 ml (2 tsp) poppy seeds to the dressing. Lemon dressing: Use freshly squeezed lemon juice instead of the vinegar. Soy sauce dressing: Mix together some chopped fresh root ginger, 1 clove crushed garlic, 15 ml (1 tbsp) sunflower or sesame oil, 15 ml (1 tbsp) dry sherry, 15 ml (1 tbsp) soy sauce and a pinch of sugar. Spicy dressing: Add 1 clove crushed garlic and a pinch of chilli powder. Use white vinegar instead of wine vinegar. Mayonnaise dressing: Use 30 ml (2 tbsp) mayonnaise instead of the oil. Herb dressing: Add 30 ml (2 tbsp) chopped fresh herbs, such as basil or mint.

---

260 Kcal/1089 KJ • 1.0 g Protein • 4.0 g Carbohydrate, of which: 3.3 g sugars •
26.9 g Fat, of which: 3.7 g saturates • trace Sodium • no Dietary Fibre

CAJUN SPICE MIX

Suitable for fish or chicken.

1.25 ml ($^1/_4$ tsp) chilli powder
15 ml (1 tbsp) paprika
15 ml (1 tbsp) ground cumin
10 ml (2 tsp) ground black pepper
15 ml (1 tbsp) dried oregano

Mix all the ingredients together. Coat fish or meat in the mixture. Cook under the grill or on the barbecue. Lightly brush with oil during cooking.

WEST INDIES MARINADE RUB

Suitable for all meats.

15 ml (1 tbsp) curry powder
15 ml (1 tbsp) ground cumin
1.25 ml ($^1/_4$ tsp) chilli powder
7.5 ml ($^1/_2$ tbsp) ground black pepper
15 ml (1 tbsp) paprika
2.5 ml ($^1/_2$ tsp) ground mixed spice

Mix all the ingredients together. Coat meat in the mixture. Cook under the grill or on the barbecue. Lightly brush with oil during cooking.

SPECIAL DISHES FOR ENTERTAINING

FISH STEW

15 ml (1 tbsp) olive oil
1 onion, peeled and diced
3 cloves garlic, crushed
8 shallots, peeled
piece of orange rind, blanched (optional)
750 g (1 1/2 lb) ripe tomatoes, skinned and roughly chopped
1 kg (2 lb) prepared fish, such as baby squid, monkfish, prawns, scallops, cod, huss
300 ml (1/2 pint) fish or vegetable stock
300 ml (1/2 pint) boiling water
sprig thyme
15–30 ml (1 – 2 tbsp) capers (optional)
60 ml (4 tbsp) chopped fresh parsley

Heat the oil in a pan and cook the onion, garlic, shallots and orange rind, if using, for about 5–7 minutes until soft. Add the tomatoes and raise the heat until they are cooked to a pulp. Lower the heat, add the fish, stock, water and thyme and bring to a simmer. Cook gently for about 15 minutes, adding the capers for the last 5 minutes. Stir in the parsley or offer separately.

208 Kcal/869 KJ • 34.1 g Protein • 6.3 g Carbohydrate, of which: 5.9 g sugars • 5.3 g Fat, of which: 0.9 g saturates • 0.3 g Sodium • 1.9 g Dietary Fibre

●

TOM YAM GUNG
(HOT AND SOUR SOUP
WITH PRAWNS)

450 g (1 lb) raw prawns with shells
900 ml (1¹/₂ pints) vegetable stock
2.5 cm (1 in) piece fresh root ginger, peeled
2 stalks lemon grass, chopped
5 dried red chillies
15 ml (1 tbsp) fish sauce (available from Asian grocers)
5 ml (1 tsp) sugar
1 onion, peeled and chopped into large pieces
100 g (4 oz) button mushrooms, cut into quarters
45 ml (3 tbsp) chopped broad-leafed parsley

Peel and devein the prawns. Heat the stock, prawn shells, ginger, lemon grass, chillies, fish sauce, sugar and onion in a saucepan. Bring to the boil and simmer for 20 minutes. Strain through a piece of muslin and return the clear liquid to a large saucepan. Add the mushrooms and prawns to the liquid and cook for 2 minutes. Add parsley, bring to the boil and serve.

64 Kcal/268 KJ • 10.7 g Protein • 3.2 g Carbohydrate, of which: 2.7 g sugars •
1.0 g Fat, of which: 0.1 g saturates • 0.7 g Sodium • 1.1 g Dietary Fibre

VENISON RAGOUT

750 g (1¹/₂ lb) venison, cut into 2.5 cm (1 in) cubes
25 ml (1 fl oz) red wine vinegar
300 ml (¹/₂ pint) good red wine, such as Bordeaux or Rioja
10 whole black peppercorns
4 juniper berries
20 ml (4 tsp) sunflower oil
2 large onions, peeled and chopped
30 ml (2 tbsp) flour
300 ml (¹/₂ pint) beef stock
10 ml (2 tsp) redcurrant jelly
100 g (3¹/₂ oz) mushrooms, quartered

Combine the venison, vinegar, 100 ml (4 fl oz) of the wine, the peppercorns and juniper berries in a large bowl. Marinate overnight or for at least 4 hours. Drain the venison, reserving the marinade, and pat dry. Heat 10 ml (2 tsp) of the oil in a pan and gently soften the onions for about 8 minutes. Remove the onions from the pan and put into a large flameproof casserole. Add the remaining oil to the pan and brown the venison in batches. Toss each completed batch in flour, then place in the casserole with the onions. When all the venison has been browned, pour the reserved marinade into the pan and bring to the boil. Remove any browned bits from the bottom of the pan. Strain and add to the casserole. Add the remaining wine, the stock and redcurrant jelly and simmer the casserole for 1 hour. Add the mushrooms and cook for at least another 30 minutes or until the meat is tender.

376 Kcal/1576 KJ • 40.3 g Protein • 13.6 g Carbohydrate, of which: 6.0 g sugars • 12.7 g Fat, of which: 4.2 g saturates • 0.1 g Sodium • 2.0 g Dietary Fibre

WEST INDIAN PORK

| 4 pork loin steaks |
| 1 portion West Indies marinade rub (see page 206) |
| sunflower oil |

Mix together all the ingredients of the West Indies marinade rub. Coat the meat in the mixture and leave for 1 hour. Heat the grill or the barbecue and when hot add the meat. Lightly brush the meat with oil and cook for 5 minutes. Turn the meat over, brush with oil and cook for a further 10 minutes.

195 Kcal/812KJ • 23.3 Protein • No Carbohydrate, of which no Sugars •
11.2 g Fat, of which: 3.6 g Saturates • 0.1 g Sodium • No Dietary Fibre

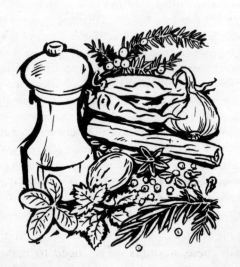

Appendix I

~ *World Health Organisation Population Nutrient Goals* * ~

Limits for population average intakes, as a percentage of daily energy/calorie intake, or in grams per day.

	Lower limit	Upper limit
Total fat	15%	**30%**
Saturated	0%	**10%**
Polyunsaturated	3%	**7%**
Dietary cholesterol	0 mg/day	300 mg/day
Total carbohydrate	**55%**	75%
Complex carbohydrates	**50%**	70%
Total dietary fibre	**27 g/day**	40 g/day
Free sugars	0	**10%**
Salt	–	**6 g/day**

* *Diet, nutrition and the prevention of chronic diseases,* World Health Organisation, 1990.

Figures in bold are the ones that as a nation we should try to achieve.
Upper limits are the most important figures relating to fats, sugar and salt. In Britain we regularly eat more than these amounts so we need to make sure that in the long-term we eat less fat, sugar and salt.

Lower limits are the most relevant for complex carbohydrates and fibre as these are the most achievable in the West. The upper figures in these categories are there so that developing countries don't move too far from their traditional diets, which supply more of these foods.

The lower limit for polyunsaturates is also important because these fats are essential for health; they have to be eaten as the body cannot synthesise them.

The zero ratings for saturated fat, cholesterol and free sugars mean these foods are not necessary for health. This is not to say that they can't be eaten ever again, but to say be careful about how much and how often.

Appendix II

~ British Government Dietary Reference Values ~

The British government's new Dietary Reference Values are similar to the WHO advice for fibre and polyunsaturated fats, but they differ a bit on saturated fat, total fat and free sugars. Some would say they are less draconian. However, WHO and the British government are unanimous on the *Eat for Life* message:
1. Eat more starchy foods, fruit and vegetables.
2. Eat less fat and free sugars

	Percentage of daily total energy/calorie intake		
	Individual minimum	Population average	Individual maximum
Total fat		33 (35)	
Saturated fat		10 (11)	
Polyunsaturates	n – 3 0.2	*6 (6.5)	10
	n – 6 1.0		
Monounsaturates		12 (13)	
**Trans fatty acids		2 (2)	
Total carbohydrate		47 (50)	
Free sugars	0	10 (11)	
Fibre (non-starch polysaccharides)	12 g/day	18 g/day	24 g/day

~ *Understanding the table* ~

The figures in brackets are for those people who do not drink alcohol, which on average accounts for five per cent of food intake. Those who don't drink can eat a little more. Protein is not mentioned, but it accounts for about 15 per cent of calories in Britain. This is much more than is needed but the British experts say it is not necessary to eat less, as it doesn't appear to do any harm at that level.

* Polyunsaturates are divided into two types: n − 3 (omega 3) and n − 6 (omega 6). Omega 3 type can be made in the body from the fatty acids found in oily fish and green leafy vegetables. Omega 6 is found in seeds and plants; the main British dietary sources are sunflower oil, corn oil and the other vegetable oils. Minimum levels have been set to prevent essential fatty acid deficiency. Most of these fatty acids can't be made in the body, and that's why they are called 'essential' fatty acids. For that reason fat cannot be cut out entirely from the diet.

** Trans fatty acids. The British line is not to eat more than we currently do − about 5 g ($^1/_4$ oz) a day each, or two per cent of total calories. They are found in cakes, biscuits, vegetable spreads, meat products and milk products. Trans fatty acids develop due to the process of hydrogenation (hardening) of fats to make them more stable and increase shelf-life of foods. Such food processing has led to an increase in trans fatty acid intake. Interest in trans fatty acids has grown because it's been suggested they may be linked to heart disease.

However, studies have failed to confirm any link between trans fatty acids and heart disease.

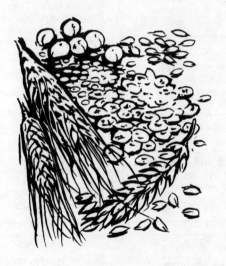

Appendix III

~ *The Benefits of Exercise* ~

Physiological functions and capacities that improve with regular exercise are on the left, and the various diseases and conditions that are influenced favourably by these changes are on the right.

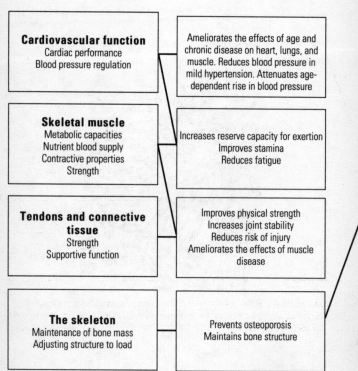

Cardiovascular function Cardiac performance Blood pressure regulation	Ameliorates the effects of age and chronic disease on heart, lungs, and muscle. Reduces blood pressure in mild hypertension. Attenuates age-dependent rise in blood pressure
Skeletal muscle Metabolic capacities Nutrient blood supply Contractive properties Strength	Increases reserve capacity for exertion Improves stamina Reduces fatigue
Tendons and connective tissue Strength Supportive function	Improves physical strength Increases joint stability Reduces risk of injury Ameliorates the effects of muscle disease
The skeleton Maintenance of bone mass Adjusting structure to load	Prevents osteoporosis Maintains bone structure

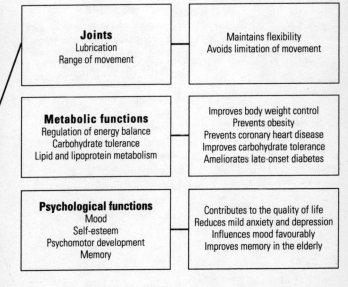

Joints
Lubrication
Range of movement

Maintains flexibility
Avoids limitation of movement

Metabolic functions
Regulation of energy balance
Carbohydrate tolerance
Lipid and lipoprotein metabolism

Improves body weight control
Prevents obesity
Prevents coronary heart disease
Improves carbohydrate tolerance
Ameliorates late-onset diabetes

Psychological functions
Mood
Self-esteem
Psychomotor development
Memory

Contributes to the quality of life
Reduces mild anxiety and depression
Influences mood favourably
Improves memory in the elderly

Diet, nutrition and the prevention of chronic diseases, World Health Organisation, 1990. Adapted from Bassey et al. Reasons for Advising Exercise, Practitioner 231:1605-1610 (1987)

~ *Index* ~